Foolproof Birth Control

BOOKS BY LAWRENCE LADER

1955
Margaret Sanger and the Fight for Birth Control

1961
The Bold Brahmins: New England's War Against Slavery,
    1831-1863

1966
Abortion

1969
Margaret Sanger: Pioneer of Birth Control (Juvenile)
    With Milton Meltzer

1971
Breeding Ourselves to Death

1972
Foolproof Birth Control: Male and Female Sterilization

Lawrence Lader has had a unique career as both author and crusader in the fields of birth control, abortion, and population control for almost twenty years.

His biography of Margaret Sanger, called by *Harper's Magazine* "an absorbing and impressive book," was followed by an exhaustive study of New England abolitionism, *The Bold Brahmins.* In 1966 the publication of *Abortion* broke down a wall of secrecy and hypocrisy which had hidden that subject for over a hundred years, and helped launch the campaign for legalized abortion that has liberalized laws in eighteen states.

Mr. Lader became volunteer chairman of the National Association for Repeal of Abortion Laws, a militant nationwide coalition, and served as chairman of the public relations committee of the Association for Voluntary Sterilization and as board member of Zero Population Growth, Inc.

A former president of the Society of Magazine Writers, he has contributed hundreds of articles to national publications, including *American Heritage, Look,* the *New York Times* Magazine, and *Reader's Digest,* and is Adjunct Associate Professor of Journalism at New York University.

FOOLPROOF BIRTH CONTROL

Male and Female Sterilization

Edited and with
Commentary by
LAWRENCE LADER

Beacon Press   Boston

Copyright © 1972 by Lawrence Lader

Library of Congress catalog number: 74-179148

International Standard Book Number: 0-8070-2182-2

Beacon Press books are published under the auspices
of the Unitarian Universalist Association

Published simultaneously in Canada by Saunders of Toronto, Ltd.

Printed in the United States of America

ACKNOWLEDGMENTS

The most devoted help has been given me in the preparation of this book by the Association for Voluntary Sterilization, 14 West 40 St., New York, N.Y. This remarkably creative and efficient organization has always been in the forefront of voluntary sterilization progress. I particularly want to thank Dr. Joseph Davis, its president; Dr. Helen Edey, chairman of the executive committee; Mr. Hugh Moore, a former president and leader in the population control movement; and Dr. Curtis Wood, its medical consultant and pioneer in voluntary sterilization.

Of the AVS staff, Mr. John Rague, executive director, and Mr. Donald Higgins, director of public relations, have been unstinting in giving time and counsel. Mrs. Evelyn Bryant and Mrs. Sally Siegel made constant contributions.

The research facilities of the Population Council in New York were put completely at my disposal, and I am deeply grateful to Dr. Christopher Tietze and Sarah Lewit for their help and encouragement.

I also want to thank Dr. Lonny Myers of the Midwest Population Center in Chicago; Dr. Matthew Freund of New York Medical College; Dr. Robert Neuwirth of Bronx-Lebanon Hospital; and Mr. Kenneth Phillips of New York for their special contributions; and Mr. and Mrs. Charles Hedberg of Westhampton Beach, N.Y., whose voluntary sterilization program should be a national model. I owe very personal gratitude to Mrs. Roberta Pryor of International Famous Agency; Mr. Ray Bentley of Beacon Press; and my wife, Joan Summers Lader.

Contents

Foolproof Birth Control

VOLUNTARY STERILIZATION: THE NEW BIRTH CONTROL

By Lawrence Lader

The emergence of voluntary sterilization as a prime method of birth control represents one of the fascinating phenomena of our time. Vasectomy, or male sterilization, is simple, safe, and inexpensive surgery that can be done in a doctor's office in fifteen minutes or so. Tubal ligation, the most common female procedure, requires hospitalization, but new techniques are reducing it to a morning's out-patient clinic surgery at modest cost. The striking advantage of voluntary sterilization is that it is permanent and virtually foolproof — attributes so desired by the public that the recent trend to VS has come close to a stampede.

The surge of sterilizations in the last two years has exceeded the most optimistic projections. In 1970, the Association for Voluntary Sterilization (AVS) estimated 100,000 procedures. But the most recent, national study, made by the medical research firm of Lea, Inc., now sets the annual number of vasectomies alone at about 750,000. Since the proportion of vasectomies to female VS runs 3 to 1, AVS believes the annual rate may reach a million.

A dominant factor in this rise from obscurity to national prominence has been AVS's public information campaign. Its speakers appeared on an average of 10 radio and television shows a month in 1966; now they are booked on at least 40 a month. The outburst of magazine articles — Life, Look, Good Housekeeping, Reader's Digest, to mention a few — has reached flood proportions. After prominent figures like Arthur Godfrey publicly announced their own vasectomies, many individuals abandoned the old tradition of secrecy and described the personal advantages of sterilization in the pages of national publications. AVS has sold thousands of sterilization pins in recent months, which men and women wear as badges of honor. When a Michigan woman staged a "Vasectomy Party" to celebrate her husband's operation, their associates in the

Zero Population Growth movement adopted the event in other states.

What has taken place is an almost overnight revolution in public and medical opinion. Strangely, voluntary sterilization was pretty well ostracized until a few years ago. Although the procedure has long been legal in every state at the choice of man or woman (Utah alone requiring medical cause), medical societies and hospitals continued to maintain a bureaucratic tangle of obstacles and restrictions against it. The very word sterilization was often shunned by the public. The wall of taboos remained so unyielding that the only national organization in the field disguised its purpose as the Human Betterment Association, and did not change its name to Association for Voluntary Sterilization until 1964.

Vasectomy was even confused with castration, and many people believed it could deprive a man not only of his sexual potency but his physical and emotional drive. Similarly, female sterilization was often thought to diminish a woman's femininity.

By all medical and psychological tests, these beliefs are baseless. Vasectomy, or the cutting of the "vas" tube in the scrotum, simply prevents sperm cells from reaching the seminal fluid, and thus eliminates them from the ejaculate. (The sperm disintegrates; the ingredients are reabsorbed into the body.) As medical studies demonstrate, in later chapters, vasectomy causes absolutely no effect on sexual potency, hormones, glands, or any other male characteristic. Nor does the tying off of the fallopian tubes for female sterilization affect any aspect of a woman's sexual or biological life.

In fact, both male and female VS often improve potency and emotional stability. By removing the trauma of unwanted pregnancy and possible contraceptive failure that freezes the emotional reactions of so many people, sterilization may produce a spontaneity and freedom in love-making that many couples have never known. Further, it eliminates some practical disadvantages of standard contraception: the possible expulsion of an intrauterine device (IUD), the clumsy insertion of a diaphragm at an inopportune moment, the unaesthetic qualities of creams and jellies, the Damoclean sword of forgetfulness that hangs over every woman on a daily regimen of pills.

The first step in the revolution, of course, was to convert the medical profession. Medical organizations (although fortunately not all doctors) seemed to demand a God-like omnipotence over the decisions of their patients, including the right of a man or woman to choose sterilization. Although the old barriers against contraception had been broken down decades before, medical policy still clung to the concept that sterilization was different, and that the patient didn't have the wisdom to terminate his or her fertility by individual choice.

To enforce this taboo, medical societies, particularly the American College of Obstetricians and Gynecologists, established rigid age-parity formulas. One typical formula required a woman 25 years of age to have borne 5 children before she could be approved for sterilization — a woman of 30 to have 4 children, a woman of 35, three.

Most hospitals applied the ACOG formula through a bureaucratic anachronism, the Abortion and Sterilization Committee (linking two disparate procedures for no logical reason). Such committees, rarely including a woman physician, sat in judgment on a patient's request for sterilization. Unless the patient met the ACOG formula, she had little chance of approval. A Catholic physician on the committee (opposed to sterilization on religious grounds) made approval even more difficult. Thus, until recently, women were trapped both in a bureaucratic maze and a medical philosophy that promoted large families as official policy. The individual's right to limit her family through sterilization was simply ignored.

Fortunately, the male applicant could avoid this bureaucracy and only had to find a urologist or surgeon willing to do vasectomy in his office. In many cities and towns this became a difficult search, although AVS has always maintained a list of about 1,600 cooperating doctors. Even in 1971, however, a Zero Population Growth officer in Dallas was so disturbed at local obstacles to vasectomy that he established a referral service (including abortion referrals), called OASIS.

Possibly the greatest single blow against these medical blocks was the U.S. Supreme Court decision of 1965 in the *Griswold* case. It not only overthrew Conecticut's anti-birth-control law, but affirmed the right of contraception and its protection under the Bill of Rights "against all governmental invasions 'of the sanctity of a man's home and the privacies of life.' "

Reasonably enough, most people concluded that a medical society or hospital could no more interfere with the right of birth control than a state government, and that sterilization — simply a lasting form of birth control — was just as much a part of family limitation as the diaphragm or pill. The *Griswold* decision, therefore, gave an immeasurable boost to the acceptance of VS, and the growing public demand to control fertility through any technique, including abortion.

The rise of the neo-feminist movement in the next few years intensified this demand. As the most aggressive proponents of the right of a woman to decide whether or not she wanted to bear a child, the National Organization for Women, Women's Liberation, and similar groups demanded absolute freedom of choice in abortion, sterilization, or other techniques. The feminists were particularly incensed that some forms of birth control — especially the Pill and its potential side effects — could endanger a woman's physical and emotional health. Why shouldn't the male assume equal responsibility in preventing pregnancy? What better method of protection than vasectomy? The espousal of vasectomy, particularly for a couple who have decided against further children, soon became a key feminist plank.

The convergence of all these forces coincided with the reorganization of AVS. When Hugh Moore, a wealthy retired manufacturer and veteran birth control campaigner, became AVS president in 1964, he quickly gave it a solid financial base, and concentrated its activities on the medical profession. Dr. H. Curtis Wood, Jr., a Philadelphia obstetrician and sterilization pioneer, was appointed medical director, travelling constantly to lecture at medical societies and hospitals as well as on radio and television. A roster of noted physicians, including Dr. Joseph Davis, now AVS president, and Dr. Helen Edey, its chairman, were added to the lecture team.

With this mounting campaign, the old medical policies began to crumble. In 1968, The Journal of the American Medical Association gave its editorial endorsement to vasectomy as "safe, quick, effective, and legal." Planned Parenthood-World Population that same year supported voluntary sterilization as part of its birth control program. In 1970, the American College of Obstetricians and Gynecologists abandoned its age-parity formula. A patient requesting sterilization now needed no other approval than the agreement of her physician.

Equally important, the U.S. Department of Health, Education and Welfare approved Medicaid payments for VS in most states. Blue Cross-Blue Shield extended coverage to VS in most insurance policies. To meet the soaring demand for vasectomy, AVS initially financed and supported the first out-patient clinic at New York's Margaret Sanger Research Bureau in 1969. Within two years over 175 out-patient clinics had been started throughout the country, 82 at hospitals.

The most concentrated opposition to the acceptance of voluntary sterilization remains the Roman Catholic Church. Still, the vast upheaval among lay Catholics in the last decade, and their increasing utilization of contraception despite Church dogma, has also affected lay attitudes towards VS. About a third of all applicants to AVS for sterilization have listed themselves as Catholics. And AVS board and committee members include such prominent Catholics as Dr. John Rock of Boston, one of the developers of the birth control pill.

Since some hospitals still cling to age-parity formulas and other obstructionist devices (and Catholic hospitals, even when receiving public funds, ban all sterilization), AVS with the American Civil Liberties Union has developed a new campaign in the courts. Six lawsuits, based on a denial of a woman's Constitutional rights, have been brought against hospitals refusing sterilization applicants. Three hospitals, including a Catholic-oriented municipal hospital receiving public money, finally agreed to accept these cases. In association with Zero Population Growth chapters, which constantly investigate obstructive policies in their areas, AVS has enlarged its campaign throughout the country.

To a great extent these breakthroughs result from a new public maturity in its concept of contraception. We have reached the point where we no longer think of it as simply the daily prevention of pregnancy. Many of us have expanded our vision to the necessity of a stable and permanent form of controlling family size. Part of this maturity stems from dissatisfaction with standard techniques: the side-effects and other potential damage from the Pill, the failure rate of IUD's, the inability of many couples to use regular methods effectively. In addition, the highly touted, "ideal contraceptive" (a safe, long-lasting, reversible injection, for example, with no impact on the biochemical system) seems little closer to realization than five years ago. Even the rapid liberalization of abortion laws offers no permanent solution. A woman with a history of contraceptive failure may not want to expose herself to repeated abortion.

As a result, an increasing segment of the public demands the security and freedom of permanent birth control as opposed to daily contraception. A new pattern in family limitation has emerged: the couple who decide at a fairly early age that it has achieved all the children it wants. Not long ago, the typical applicants for sterilization were a husband aged forty and a wife of thirty-five or so who had three or four children and considered themselves too old to raise more. Today, a growing segment of VS applicants are under thirty, some under twenty-five. Once determined to limit their families to one or two children (or none, in some cases), they quickly grasp the advantages of sterilization over twenty or more years of incessant contraceptive fears and problems.

The impact of the population crisis and environmental damage in the last few years has sharply increased the growth of this concept. In addition to personal motivations for early sterilization, we now have the added factor of social responsibility. A couple committed to population control and the small family often want to strengthen this commitment with its own guarantee against unwanted fertility. This combination of personal and social goals accounts for the crusading zeal of many couples who wear sterilization pins, extol the virtues of VS among their friends, and are increasingly adopting un- wanted children.

"Once you've reached the family size you want, the only sane choice for a couple which feels deeply about popu- lation control is to avoid any possible risk of unwanted preg- nancy," concludes Charles Hedberg, a father of two and ZPG leader from Suffolk County, New York, who recently had a vasectomy. "We've learned that sterilization can be one of the most satisfying and constructive steps a family can make."

With all its advantages, however, VS cannot be treated as a universal panacea. While most studies indicate a high percentage of satisfaction among men and women, an occa- sional case chooses VS for the wrong reasons, expecting it to solve sexual maladjustments and other deeply rooted personal problems. Physicians with long experience in sterilization stress that the decision must be weighed carefully. Usually they interview an applicant at length — both husband and wife in the case of marriage. Often they ask the applicant to con- sider the decision for a week, or a month, before undergoing surgery.

VS must still be held an irreversible procedure. No matter how convinced an applicant is of its necessity, he must still ponder a range of future possibilities. If either spouse dies, if any or all present children are killed in an accident, or even if the couple is divorced, would the applicant ever seek remarriage and further offspring?

Such critical issues, however, may lose their importance with the advance of medical research. Under traditional methods of vasectomy, studies show that successful restora- tion of fertility has been achieved in up to 40 per cent of all cases. (The reversal rate of female tubal ligation is about 40 per cent.) Now the prime target of researchers has become a guaranteed-reversible technique of vasectomy; perhaps a tiny valve implanted in the vas in the "off" position, which Drs.

Joseph E. Davis and Matthew Freund of New York Medical College are ready to test on males after successful animal studies. If at any time the man decides he wants to father another child, the valve can be turned on to allow the flow of sperm.

As a back-up technique for standard vasectomy or the new valve implants, Dr. Freund and other researchers are close to perfecting "sperm banks." Before undergoing vasectomy, a man who may want to father a child at some future date would simply deposit a supply of sperm at a hospital or clinic "bank." There, it would be kept frozen and in permanently usable state for years. If the man and his wife ever decide on another child, the sperm can be introduced into her vagina to produce the desired pregnancy through artificial insemination.

These research breakthroughs could soon bring voluntary sterilization to a climactic stage. With a guaranteed-reversible valve, vasectomy would have the supreme advantage of permanence, simplicity, safety, and low cost — and still retain the attributes of standard contraception by allowing the man to restore his fertility with a brief trip to the doctor's office. Aesthetically, it would probably rank over most present birth control methods. Psychologically, it could be a boon to women who have increasingly insisted that the male take over contraceptive responsibility. Voluntary sterilization, only a few years ago the maligned stepchild of family planning and population control, could eventually become their savior.

Part One ☿♂

Advantages of Voluntary Sterilization: Forces Behind the Rising Demand

1 FOOLPROOF BIRTH CONTROL

by Ernest Dunbar

Mr. and Mrs. David Braum, a childless couple, had a problem. She had been taking a birth-control pill for three years, and her gynecologist felt that was too long. The pair had tried other contraceptive methods but were turned off by them. "It kills the spontaneity of the sex act," Braum says. He had other reservations: "I decided a long time ago, I guess when I was 18, that most people had children for the wrong reasons — for ego involvement or for property reasons, to have somebody to pass your property on to." Now 26 and an assistant director of purchasing at New York's Maimonides Medical Center, David Braum says, "Two years in the Army in Vietnam solidified my thinking. I decided I didn't want to provide any more bodies for the Establishment to staff armies with." He'd also met another G.I. who had had a vasectomy, the male sterilization operation.

So, with his wife's approval, Braum decided to have a vasectomy. He applied to the Association for Voluntary Sterilization,* a New York-based organization, for the name of a doctor who would perform the operation. AVS is a 33-year-old agency, funded through private contributions, whose mission is to stimulate public interest in voluntary sterilization. The Association maintains a directory of some 1,600 cooperating U.S. physicians who will perform sterilization surgery on men and women referred to them by AVS. In 1960, 60 percent of those applying to AVS were women. Today, about 75 percent of the referrals are men. Braum chose Dr. Philip R. Roen, a Manhattan physician, who spent part of a one-hour screening interview trying to dissuade the couple because they had no children. "But," says Braum, "when he saw we were serious, he said OK." Last April, David Braum went to Dr. Roen's offices, and in minutes the surgery was done. The operation cost $200, about 80 percent of which was covered by Braum's medical insurance.

Ten days later, he was certified sperm-free. "Now the anxiety is zero," he says, "the anxiety that is always present with the pill." He adds, with a laugh, "It's like those deodorant ads say: 'It takes the worry out of being close!' "

For Richard Sampson, 35, a New Jersey airline pilot, a vasectomy was the logical solution to a dilemma that troubled his marriage. He and his wife have three children, and Mary Jane Sampson has a spinal ailment that further pregnancies could aggravate. She had encountered difficulties with the pill. Her husband, a veteran of eight and a half years in the U.S. Air Force, had met many men in the service who had had vasectomies, and they recommended the operation to him. In March of 1969, he called the Association's referral service for the name of a local doctor. The urologist interviewed them for 45 minutes on a Tuesday. The following Friday, they returned for the surgery, which took 25 minutes. The cost: $100. Looking back on the experience two years later, Sampson says, "There's no doubt about it, it adds to your marriage. It even enters into the rest of your family life. I recommend it for people who feel they've had enough kids."

*For information, write to 14 West 40th St., New York, N.Y. 10018.

The Braums and the Sampsons are part of a growing trend toward vasectomy, an operation that helps couples limit births and may tone up tense marriages in the process. Men whose wives have experienced harmful side effects with birth-control pills, or who feel that other forms of contraception take the fun out of sex are flocking to physicians for sterilization. Most such men and their wives report that the result of the operation is a happier, more pleasureful marital relationship.

The vasectomy is a simple surgical procedure that involves severing the two tubes that carry the sperm. In an operation usually carried out in a doctor's office under local anesthesia, a half-inch incision is made on both sides of the scrotum, each tube (*vas deferens*) is lifted out and a small section removed. The tubes are then closed off. Sperm continue to be produced but are resorbed by the body instead of going into the seminal fluid. That's the only change. A man continues to ejaculate semen, but the fluid contains no sperm. The operation takes 15 to 30 minutes and, in most cases, the patient may return to work the next day. Unlike female sterilization, which requires hospitalization and is regarded as major surgery, the vasectomy is walk-in, walk-out simplicity. The operation is covered by Blue Cross, Blue Shield and Medicaid in most states.

While vasectomies have been performed in small numbers until recently, the operation has been enmeshed in controversy and ignorance, even within the medical profession itself.

Dr. Joseph E. Davis, a urologist and an assistant professor of urology at New York Medical College, says: "The operation used to be frowned upon in the profession. Some doctors opposed it on moral grounds, others thought it illegal." Actually, the operation is legal in all 50 states, though Utah specifies that there must be a medical necessity. A similar law in Connecticut has been repealed, effective in October, 1971. The Roman Catholic Church opposes the operation as a form of birth control. "I attended a meeting recently here in New York," adds Dr. Davis, "and did not meet one young urologist who was not doing vasectomies. Ironically, many of these urologists from New Jersey and other nearby points used to send me their patients because they didn't want to do this surgery!"

John R. Rague, executive director of the Association for Voluntary Sterilization, confirms the new interest in vas surgery. He estimates that more than 100,000 men had vasectomies in 1970, and that there are now two million men of procreative age in the U.S. who have had the operation. [Revised to 750,000 and three million — Ed.]

The takeoff point for male sterilization came in 1969, according to Rague. "We offered a grant to any hospital in the city of New York that would open a vasectomy clinic," he says. "Our medical consultant visited, phoned or wrote every hospital in town, and not a single one accepted. Then we gave a $30,000 grant to the Margaret Sanger Research Bureau, a fertility and anti-fertility agency, and a Sanger vasectomy clinic was started." The Sanger clinic began doing the operations at the rate of four to eight a week, on Friday afternoons so that patients could have the weekend to recuperate. Following publicity about the new facility, inquiries poured in, and Sanger is now doing 15 to 20 vasectomies a week on an expanded schedule. Since October, 1969, when the service was begun, more than 450 have been performed and there is a waiting list of over 150. [Revised to 760 and 100 — Ed.]

At Sanger, a married applicant is interviewed with his wife by a psychiatrist, who probes to find out if the couple have considered all the ramifications of the operation. What if the wife should die, or if they are divorced and the husband remarries? What if their present children should die? What if . . . ? Single applicants are checked to see if they have psychiatric problems and if they are unalterably committed to a childless future. When the psychiatrist approves, there is still a waiting period of about a month before the surgery is done. The Sanger clinic charges up to $150 for the service, depending upon the applicant's ability to pay.

With the success of the Sanger clinic demonstrating a

demand, other agencies entered the field. Several New York hospitals have begun vasectomy services. The Planned Parenthood Federation has opened ten similar clinics around the nation, and hopes to have 25 going by the end of 1971.

Norman Fleishman, executive director of Planned Parenthood in Los Angeles, calls vasectomy "the most underrated form of birth control in America." He himself has had the operation. Before coming to Los Angeles, Fleishman started a Planned Parenthood vas clinic in Houston, against strong local opposition. "When I came to Houston, you could hardly get one," he recalls. "It was worse than an abortion. Now, the Houston clinic is doing 36 a week and there is a six-week backlog." In Los Angeles, the Planned Parenthood agency has persuaded ten physicians to perform the surgery for as little as $50 for those who can't afford the usual fee. Other doctors do it for $90. "We are referring 100 men a week," Fleishman says, "and the number is steadily going up."

Dr. Eugene Mathias, a Los Angeles surgeon who has done over 5,000 vasectomies in the past 25 years, says, "The demand is growing by leaps and bounds. I performed twice as many operations in 1970 as I did in 1969. I'm situated close to the Douglas, Northrop and Lockheed aviation plants, and many of their workers come in for vas surgery. Most of them say, 'Ye Gods, if I'd known it was this simple, I'd have come in years ago!' " Like many other private surgeons who perform vasectomies, Dr. Mathias has a one-month backlog of applicants. In California, the operation has been performed much more frequently than in the East, but the gap is narrowing.

While the popularity of the vasectomy soars, physicians still disagree about who can — and should — get the surgery. With certain exceptions, unmarried men under 28 and childless couples who have not been married very long have been turned down at Sanger clinic. On the other hand, Dr. Joseph E. Davis, who operates at Sanger, has less severe rules in his private practice. "I take a very liberal line," he says. "If you have a 23-year-old guy with a 19-year-old wife, who've already had four kids, if he makes $5,000 a year and they can't use the pill, I think a vasectomy should be done. I don't think doctors should play God. If the couple know what the ramifications are, they should be allowed to have the operation." The Association for Voluntary Sterilization also takes a less rigid line. John Rague says, "Our policy is that a man or a woman has the right to the use of his own body. We agree with the American College of Obstetricians and Gynecologists, which has ruled sterilization should be available to any competent adult. If the applicant is 21 and sane, regardless of his marital status or number of children, we will refer him to a willing physician."

But Dr. William L. F. Ferber, another New York urologist, will not go quite so far. "I personally reserve this operation for people who are married," he says. "I'm aware that in many places, especially California, they will sterilize any bachelor who asks, but I don't." On the other hand, Dr. Mathias in Los Angeles says simply, "I try to make it available as liberally as possible." The American Medical Association has not issued a policy statement on the operation but at least one AMA *Journal* editorial has described vasectomies as safe, simple and legal.

In Houston, the Planned Parenthood clinic will perform the surgery on the same day that an applicant comes in, and does not require the wife to be present at the preoperative interview. But Sanger clinic doctors and many private physicians insist on extensive talk with husband and wife, and both are usually asked to sign a release form. The reasons are many: Sometimes a wife may press the surgery on a reluctant husband; sometimes a spouse may seek the operation as a solution for impotency problems (which it isn't); in other instances, men may undergo the operation with the expectancy that it can be reversed later. Though surgeons can now rejoin the severed vas in many cases, most doctors tell patients that the operation is irreversible.

Apart from the negligible physical discomfort, a vasectomy can involve certain psychological risks that preoperative counseling by the physician helps avoid. Dr. Elliot

Leiter, an associate professor of urology at New York's Mt. Sinai, says, "No matter how rationally a man accepts the fact that cutting his vas interferes with none of his sexual functions — his potency, his erections, his ability to consummate intercourse, his orgasms, that all it does is eradicate the sperm in his semen — there's hardly a man who doesn't have some kind of psychological hang-up about sexual function."

Dr. Matthew Freund, a New York physiologist, agrees. "It takes a certain amount of self-knowledge and psychological stability to undergo this," he observes. "You would not expect someone who feels sexually challenged to have an operation on his genital area." Freund, who has studied the physiological performances of couples after the husband has had a vasectomy, says, "A substantial number felt their sex life was better, that the freedom they now experienced led to more sexual pleasure. While the actual frequency of sexual relations remained about the same, there was a definitely marked *perception* of an improved sex life, a *feeling* of improvement."

Formerly, few men who had had a vasectomy were willing to acknowledge it, but the increasing popularity of the operation and a concurrent shift toward candor among younger people have enabled couples like the Braums and Sampsons to discuss their experience with others.

Ken Phillips, a 31-year-old educator with three children, says, "It comes up all the time at cocktail parties. One of the biggest fears people have comes from not knowing what it's really like. I tell them it didn't affect my ego or my drives and that sex now is a lot more enjoyable."

Mary Jane Sampson says wives she knows are often curious. "They won't come right out and ask," she says with a grin. "They sort of smile and make little jokes, but they are anxious to know about it. What they really want to know is, 'What are your marital relations like after that?' There is still a lack of information about the operation among the public, and people feel a little intimidated and embarrassed about wanting to know."

Planned Parenthood's Norman Fleishman tells of an employee at the Disney Studios who put the excised sections of his tubes into a plastic cube that he wears on his key chain: "During lulls at cocktail parties, he'd explain what it was. Now, 14 of his Disney co-workers have had vasectomies!"

Until the last few years, most of the applicants for sterilization came from upper-income, better-educated groups, including many physicians. As the satisfied patients spread the word, the pattern is changing. The Sanger clinic director, Dr. Aquiles Sobrero, says: "At the beginning, we got mostly white-collar workers, doctors, professors and so forth. Now, the picture is mixed. We are servicing almost anyone, including a large number of policemen." He adds that a lot of younger men who don't want children are having the operation. There are also men "who have been using contraceptives for ten to fifteen years." John Rague says, "The people we refer to physicians cut across all classes, from Ph.D.'s to illiterates. There are a lot of young people who are pessimistic about the future of this biosphere, or who feel that children don't fit into the new lifestyle. They don't feel the pressure to have them that older generations did. 'If we want them, we'll adopt them,' they say."

Dr. Davis, who does "between 50 and 60" vasectomies a month (privately and at Sanger), says, "Most of my private patients are in their late 30's, with two or three children. The wife has been on the pill and they've tried other forms of contraception. I have white middle-class, black middle-class, Chinese middle-class and an occasional poor person."

Davis feels the poor who want vas surgery are disadvantaged. "We've had a big fight with the city of New York to get them to allow vasectomies in city hospitals. In spite of the fact that female sterilization is being done all the time, a couple of hospitals have refused to do vasectomies!"

Nonetheless, official attitudes toward the operation are changing, reflecting the growing demand.

Last May, the Department of Defense revised its regulations to permit vasectomies for servicemen at military hospitals under more liberal guidelines, and regardless of local laws on sterilization. One serviceman who got the operation soon after the rule revision was a 25-year-old Air Force lieutenant. He and his wife wished to remain childless.

As enthusiasm for the male operation spreads, men who have had vas surgery are less frequently viewed.as eunuchs by their neighbors. Says Richard Sampson, "I was playing golf recently with a man whose wife had just had a baby but was not feeling her old self after the child was born. They have four 'stair-step' kids. I mentioned to him that I'd had a vasectomy and told him what it involved. Ten minutes after I got home from the golf course, the phone rang. He wanted to know the name of my doctor!"

2   BIRTH CONTROL FOR MEN

by Evan McLeod Wylie

Even for the most determined, disciplined and well-informed couples, birth control by any of the current contraception methods is burdensome and carries with it an element of risk. Indeed, of the 3,500,000 births in the United States each year, roughly one third are estimated to be "unplanned." Little wonder that interest is growing rapidly in the least expensive and most reliable form of contraception, the male sterilization operation called vasectomy.

"For millions of American families of all economic levels, this method provides the only sure means of limiting family size to the number of children they can provide for, nurture and love," says Dr. H. Curtis Wood, Jr., a medical consultant to the Association for Voluntary Sterilization. Already an estimated one million U.S. husbands have turned to this simple, painless technique. [Revised to three million — Ed.] One father of four says, "My wife and I were having a child a year. We used contraception, but like almost everyone else we often failed to use it at the right time." For him, and for his wife, vasectomy is a "great emancipator that enhances one's pleasure by removing the fear of pregnancy."

Though doctors have been performing vasectomies for more than 50 years, many people are confused about the operation, or needlessly fearful. It is actually quite uncomplicated, and is often performed in the doctor's office.

The tiny sperm cells that fertilize the female ovum to reproduce the human species are manufactured within the male testicles, and travel by two hollow, tube-like ducts called the vas deferens to the prostate gland in the pelvic cavity. There they mix with seminal fluid and are ejected from the penis during intercourse. In the vasectomy, the surgeon snips out a small piece of each vas deferens — usually about a quarter of an inch — and ties the severed ends with surgical thread before burying them in surrounding tissue. This prevents sperm cells from traveling from the testicles to the prostate, thus rendering the seminal fluid spermless and incapable of bringing about conception. In essence, the procedure is nothing more than cutting a length of tubing in two pieces and capping the ends.

To reach the twin vas deferens tubes, the surgeon normally need make only two half-inch incisions in the skin of the upper scrotum. He uses a local anesthetic, does not have to touch any vital organ, major blood vessel, nerve trunk, bone, or heavy layer of muscle. Nor are the other parts of the male reproductive system — testicles, penis, or prostate — involved. After the operation, there are no side effects related to urination, no impairment of any normal activity. While doctors recommend 24 to 48 hours of rest following the surgery, some men return to work the next day. The only caution, really, is that it may take five or six weeks for the last lingering sperm cells to disappear, and contraceptive measures must be continued until lab tests confirm that no more sperm are present in the seminal fluid.

Vasectomy has no effect on sexual intercourse, because the male seminal fluid — the overwhelming portion of ejaculation — is 95 percent manufactured in the seminal vesicles and prostate, which are unaffected by the vasectomy. One might expect that the sperm cells, which can no longer leave the body, might cause swelling or discomfort. This does not happen. Sperm cells produced after the operation are simply reabsorbed into the body with no harmful results.

Nor does the operation affect production of the male hormones responsible for such masculine characteristics as facial beard and deeper voice. These are manufactured in the tissue spaces of the testicles *between* the tubules and absorbed directly into the bloodstream. A man remains as robust as ever.

Is there danger that a man may feel psychologically injured or "castrated" by a vasectomy? Extensive studies of men who have undergone vasectomies have uncovered few negative reactions and these only in individuals who had psychological or sexual potency problems before the operation. In one recent survey of married men, three out of four reported *more* active sex lives after vasectomy than before, and the overwhelming majority reported that their relations with their wives had improved. Meanwhile, wives have reported approval of vasectomy, because it relieves them of the necessity of taking birth-control measures.

A common query about vasectomy is: Can a man's fertility be restored? The answer is yes; reversal is possible. However, reconnecting the tiny tubes is considerably more complex than severing them, and results cannot be guaranteed. (Still in the research stage is a technique for making the vasectomy temporary and reversible by surgically inserting removable silastic plugs in the vas deferens.) Actually, physicians report that fewer than one out of 100 of their vasectomy patients have requested a reverse operation.

Obviously, sterilization via vasectomy should be undertaken only when a man is certain about his decision not to father any more children. And both husband and wife should fully agree on the desirability of the operation.

Vasectomy is surprisingly inexpensive. The surgeon's fee is generally in the $50-$250 range, with private health insurance policies paying all or a substantial portion of the bill in most states. Medicaid programs in 35 states now pay for voluntary sterilization operations.

Vasectomy is legal in all states, and the Association for Voluntary Sterilization has a roster of some 1600 physicians across the nation who perform the operation regularly. Additionally, vasectomy services have been established at Planned

Parenthood centers in a number of U.S. cities.

Only the Roman Catholic Church, among major religious groups, remains officially opposed to vasectomy, as it is to all methods of birth control except the so-called "rhythm method." But the Association for Voluntary Sterilization reports that approximately 30 percent of the private inquiries it receives about sterilization operations, including vasectomy, come from Catholics.

Proponents of voluntary sterilization point to the social benefit that vasectomy may bring to all mankind as a step toward population control. Dr. Paul Ehrlich, of Stanford University, author of *The Population Bomb,* sees vasectomy as an important key to human survival. Already, it has proved a potent factor in introducing effective birth control in India, Japan and Pakistan. At latest count, 7,100,000 Indians had obtained sterilization operations, 80 percent of them men, and vasectomy is considered the most effective population-control measure of all in that country. "Voluntary sterilization," says Dr. Sripati Chandrasekhar, former Minister of State for Family Planning in India, "will be the physical salvation of mankind."

At least 150,000 Americans [revised to 750,000 — Ed.] are expected to undergo vasectomies in 1971. There seems little doubt that the number will continue to rise as more and more of the estimated 39 million couples in this country who have two or more children learn about the operation. Until new and better methods of controlling human fertility are developed, vasectomy deserves consideration as an effective, simple, worry-free birth control measure.

3   NEW BIRTH CONTROL FREEDOM FOR WOMEN

by Evan McLeod Wylie

At eight o'clock one recent morning, Mrs. Dorothy McLean (not her real name) was rolled into an operating room in Baltimore's Johns Hopkins Hospital. Less than 48 hours earlier, she had given birth to her third child, a healthy, blue-eyed girl. Now — because she and her husband had decided that three children were as many as they could properly bring up — Mrs. McLean was scheluled for special surgery.

Thirty minutes after her operation began, Mrs. McLean was on her way to a recovery room. And three days later she was home with her baby in her arms, free forever from the prospect of an unwanted pregnancy.

Mrs. McLean's surgery is called voluntary sterilization. In the past, the procedure has been shrouded in fear and misunderstanding. But now, across the nation, hospitals and physicians are moving to make the operation readily available to all who request it. Most frequently undergone by women who, like Mrs. McLean, are still in the hospital after childbirth, it can be performed at any time except during pregnancy.

To understand what the sterilization operation is, and why it's so effective, consider briefly the female reproductive system. From the upper portion of the uterus the twin fallopian tubes branch out, leading to the two ovaries. Once monthly, from adolescence until middle age, a single ripe egg, released by one of the ovaries, is drawn into one of the fallopian tubes to begin its journey to the uterus. If, during this journey, the egg should encounter a single male sperm (several million are released during sexual intercourse), a pregnancy may take place. But if the egg and sperm cannot meet because the fallopian tubes have been blocked off from the uterus, pregnancy is impossible.

The surgical method most commonly used is called tubal ligation. First the surgeon makes an incision in the lower abdomen. Then he lifts each tube, clamps and snips out a small piece midway between the uterus and ovary and "ligates" (ties off) the severed ends with surgical sutures. The ovaries and uterus remain intact. No glands or organs are removed. No nerve trunks or major blood vessels are disturbed. A woman's femininity is not affected because her ovaries continue producing female hormones. Menstrual periods still occur, and the ovaries release a ripe egg each month (the egg in the blocked-off tube is quickly reabsorbed into the body). The operation involves no unpleasant side effects, and no further birth control precautions need be taken by a wife or her husband.

The one major disadvantage to voluntary sterilization as a birth control measure is that it *must* be considered permanent. While there is a possibility that a woman's fertility may be restored by reconnecting the tubes, success rates vary widely (from zero to 65 percent, depending on the surgical procedure that is used and the skill of the surgeon attempting the reconnection). "No woman should seek sterilization," says one doctor, "unless she is absolutely certain she wants no more children."

A woman in her 30s or 40s is usually considered an ideal candidate for sterilization, but an increasing number of physicians believe that the procedure is even more valuable for the younger woman who has completed her family and faces 20 or more years of fertility. Over such a long period, the chances of an unplanned pregnancy with other methods of birth control are much higher than generally realized. Also, as Dr. Helen Edey, of New York City, emphasizes, "Many women are dubious about the safety of taking the contraceptive pill for a long period, and perhaps rightly so. For them, sterilization is a safe, dependable alternative."

Is voluntary sterilization likely to cause harmful psychological side effects? For the woman who has made up her own mind, carefully and without coercion, the answer appears to be no. In fact, recent studies indicate that the most common reaction is a feeling of relief brought about by freedom from anxiety about unwanted pregnancy and the distractions of other birth-control methods.

Why hasn't voluntary sterilization been more common? One reason is that until recently both the public and a large segment of the medical profession have been confused about its legality. Actually, voluntary sterilization is legal in all 50 states, whether the woman is married, separated, single, widowed or divorced. (Utah and Connecticut require that the operation be performed for "medical necessity," although the Connecticut law will be changed in October [1971] to permit sterilization for "socio-economic" reasons.)

Another reason is that hospitals have generally followed recommendations on sterilization formulated by the American

College of Obstetricians and Gynecologists some years ago. These recommendations, which required that a woman bear a specific number of children and attain a certain age in order to be eligible for the operation, had no legal basis but were considered authoritative in setting hospital policies. Recently, however, ACOG liberalized its restrictive guidelines. Its new policy simply states that if sterilization is requested by the patient, and her physician agrees, no further "consultation" is required. Many hospitals are now following this lead. Says the administrator of a Wisconsin hospital which has liberalized its sterilization rules, "We exist to perform certain services — those which are permitted by law and which reflect the current feeling of society."

By contrast, hospitals and physicians who have recently refused to permit voluntary sterilization are being challenged with lawsuits filed by individual women and interested organizations. In the first case in the nation filed against a city hospital, a 38-year-old mother alleged that she requested Fordham Hospital in the Bronx, N.Y., to sterilize her while she was there for the delivery of her tenth child. The hospital refused, giving no reason except that sterilization operations were never performed there because of an "unwritten law." Within a few weeks after the lawsuit was filed, Fordham Hospital decided to permit the operation. "If a woman is a good surgical risk," observes one lawyer, "hospitals are on dubious constitutional grounds in denying her request."

How much does sterilization cost? If it is done while a woman is in the hospital for childbirth, the only additional charges are the surgeon's fee, which is about $300, and related operating-room expenses, plus charges for an extra day or so in the hospital. If a woman elects to enter the hospital specifically for sterilization, the cost would increase according to her length of stay (usually about five days). Private health-insurance plans now pay for all or part of the bill in the majority of states, and Medicaid programs in 46 states include in their benefits the cost of voluntary-sterilization operations (in 30 of these states when it is done "for any reason," in 16, when done "for medical necessity"). Advocates of sterilization point out that these costs are extremely low when compared to the expense to a family of unplanned pregnancies.

Meanwhile, new procedures which may make sterilization even less expensive are being developed. An increasing number of surgeons favor a method developed in Europe called laparoscopic tubal sterilization. Two tiny abdominal incisions are made, one at the navel, resulting in no visible scar, and the other lower down in the abdominal wall, with a scar that will be scarcely visible. First, a harmless neutral gas is instilled to distend the abdomen and, by displacing the vital organs, to facilitate observation of the fallopian tubbs. Then a hollow metal tube is inserted through which the laparoscope, a telescope-like instrument, is placed. A bright light fitted to the "scope" illuminates the interior of the abdomen and a magnifying lens improves the surgeon's vision. He then makes the second tiny incision and slips in another hollow "scope" through which he manipulates a pair of miniature electric tongs. With the tongs, he cauterizes and severs a portion of each tube adjacent to the uterus.

At New York's Downstate Medical Center, where Dr. Alvin Siegler has trained operating-room teams to perform laparoscopic tubal sterilizations in 20 minutes, the patient stays in the hospital less than two full days. In Phoenix, Ariz., laparoscopies are being done outside a hospital — in a surgicenter equipped with an operating room, provisions for anesthesia, recovery rooms and a small laboratory. The cost: about $500. At Johns Hopkins Hospital in Baltimore, where a single-incision technique with local anesthetic is being used, a laparoscopy patient is admitted in the morning and leaves for home in the afternoon.

Voluntary sterilization for women is strongly supported by advocates of birth control such as the Planned Parenthood Association, and by groups concerned about world population problems, including Zero Population Growth (ZPG). A recent Gallup poll reported that 64 percent of Americans now favor voluntary sterilization. Many religious leaders have voiced approval. Women's rights groups are organizing to tell women that the operation is legal, and to challenge resisting hospitals.

Last year, more than 200,000 women within the United States chose voluntary sterilization. As the trend toward liberalized policies in hospitals continues, the number of women seeking the operation is expected to rise sharply. Clearly — at least until better means of controlling human fertility are developed — this safe and legal method of birth control should no longer be denied to women who want it.

4 ONE GP'S PERSONAL AND PROFESSIONAL COMMITMENT

by Carl B. Erling, M.D.

What prompted the whole thing, I suppose, was seeing Stanford ecologist Paul Ehrlich on a late-night television talk-show. Both my wife, Bunnie (a former nurse whom I married the day my internship ended), and I saw that show. Dr. Ehrlich talked about how he had undergone sterilization after fathering only one child. He thinks we're heading for doomsday because the general public thinks population is someone else's problem. He "came on strong" and set us thinking.

A few days later, I picked up Ehrlich's book *The Population Bomb* at a newsstand and brought it home. We read it and were impressed.

Just a few years ago, it was difficult to find a physician who would perform a vasectomy. More recently, however, certain of my colleagues have realized their civic and medical responsibility. Ted Owens, a respected St. Paul surgeon, felt this way. By scrubbing with Ted I learned his technique, and, last spring, I began counseling my patients on vasectomy as one method of contraception. About twenty-five have asked me to perform the procedure. One of my partners has also begun doing it.

All this time, Bunnie and I were talking about a vasectomy for us. I emphasize the plural pronoun because we realized that the operation would affect both our lives. Yet, at the same time, the decision didn't seem earth-shaking to us; it was simply logical. When we married, we thought it would be ideal to have three or four children. We still feel that way, but are convinced that only two of these children should be natural and that any others should be adopted.

The alternative to a sterilization procedure, we agreed, would be twenty-five years of life with The Pill, the IUD, or some other less effective method. I didn't want my wife subjected to the potential complications of many artificial contraceptive techniques. So, the choice wasn't difficult.

Still, we put off making the actual commitment. "When are you going to make that appointment," Bunnie would say. "Oh, next week when I have a little time," I'd reply. Then we heard Paul Ehrlich again. He was speaking at the University of Minnesota, and his thoughts were even more persuasive when delivered in person. I made the appointment.

The procedure was done under local anesthesia at a hospital where I do not make rounds. The surgeon advised me to take the day off, and I did. But I kept my tennis date for the next morning and played two sets. Although I don't advise my patients to do that, it gives some idea of the minimal discomfort that is involved.

In the past ten months since my vasectomy, I have been even more pleased with our decision. I've become an exponent of zero population growth; and, as a family practitioner with a fairly active obstetrical practice, I have an ample opportunity to use my influence.

But is it right to influence my patients toward limiting their family size?

My policy is to ask childbearing women, at the time of physical examination or postpartum checkups, what form of contraception they use and if they desire additional counseling. Frequently, the patient appears relieved that I brought up the subject. I include in our discussion all the practical forms of contraception, pointing out the advantages and disadvantages of each. If the patient appears convinced that The Pill, IUD, or rhythm is for her, I don't press the point. But if she is interested in sterilization, I explain both vasectomy and tubal ligation.

Before agreeing to perform a vasectomy, I consider it mandatory to talk with both man and wife. In this way I know that both understand all the implications, and I have a chance to assess their psychological stability. The people interested in vasectomy are primarily middle-class couples with better-than-average educations. Many are professionals. Often they are younger and have two or three children already. So, the communication problems are minimal. Nevertheless, I give them a release to sign. It states that they understand what vasectomy is, what its effect will be, and absolves me if there is any pregnancy. Of course, they still might sue if the latter occurs.

I remove about an inch to an inch-and-a-quarter segment of the vas deferens, stick tie the ends with 3.0 silk sutures, and cauterize them. We check for persistent spermatozoa at one month and at six months postoperatively. The patient takes no medication postoperatively but wears an athletic supporter for a few days.

Probably the most discomforting aspect of the whole procedure occurs with the regrowth of the pubic and scrotal hair. This hair serves a real purpose in preventing the scrotum from sticking to the thighs and in disseminating sweat.

Vasectomies are only a small part of my practice, and probably always will be so. But, without making such procedures the major part of his practice, the family practitioner is in an unusually advantageous position to counsel about them. He usually knows the whole family, its medical and social background, and the individual problems it faces. But he must have a feeling for the family to recommend the correct type of contraception.

Recently, I've begun speaking to small groups in schools and elsewhere about the population problem. This takes away some free evenings, but I feel a responsibility that is both personal and professional.

My practice involves mostly middle-class citizens where the population problem is primarily centered. Physicians could make vasectomies more available to other socioeconomic groups by promoting vasectomy counseling in established planned-parenthood clinics. In such clinics, the operation should be arranged without regard for the patient's ability to pay. Criteria should be confined to age, psychological soundness, and an awareness of all the ramifications of sterilization.

Coercion in any form must never become part of population control. But if Americans are given the facts and the opportunity to practice effective contraception, I believe they will act responsibly.

5   ONE COUPLE'S DECISION

by Kenneth H. Phillips

A 31-year-old educational planning and fund-raising specialist at the Institute of International Education in New York City, Kenneth H. Phillips graduated from Princeton University, received his Master's degree in English from the University of Michigan, and is now working towards a Ph.D. in economics from New York University. He had his vasectomy in May 1969.

Shortly after Belinda told me she was unexpectedly pregnant with our third child, we began to gather information about sterilization. We didn't want any more children and felt, in fact, that two were really enough. We believed this because of the broad social implications of world population growth and our deeply felt personal convictions about the quality and style of family life.

The prospective doubling, tripling, and quadrupling of population took on a real meaning for us through our own children (Karlton 7, Tania 4, and Larissa 2) who will be young adults in 2000 and whose children could well greet the 22nd century! The unendurable traffic jams, air pollution, deteriorating public services, disappearing personal freedom, and vanishing open spaces are reason enough to stop producing more children; the signs of food riots, plagues, and mass starvation in the developing world should convince any who persist in wanting a large family. Quite bluntly, it is immoral to produce a large family today.

It is also impractical. While the population problem was a factor in our decision, our own family life and hopes for our personal future argued most persuasively for strict and 100% certain limitation on family size. Children are bundles of potential. Like vast reservoirs waiting to be filled, they can take in information and experiences far faster than any parents can provide them (even when supplemented by "Sesame Street," good schools, and other special programs). With more than one or two children, parents simply cannot develop the children's full potential, cannot keep up with their needs, cannot retain the flexibility and capability to seek an essential variety of experiences for them. In our world, where education, broadly defined, is the means for a person's success (however he defines it) and for his own personal happiness and achievement, only the wealthy can afford the external costs of several children. But even for them, they remain only two parents with only 24 hours a day; and hired maids and older siblings are no substitutes. Our personal choice was to limit our family so we could make more of it.

But even if parents want a larger family (or change their minds about sterilization), there are better ways of expanding family size than simple reproduction. Adoption is the most obvious and effective — and most urgently needed. Temporary foster child care or summertime Fresh Air Fund arrangements are also available. Having a foreign student stay in one's home has many advantages. These alternatives to large families provide important social benefits to all the participants as well as relieving some of the most pressing problems facing us.

With these thoughts in mind, my wife and I wanted to stop producing babies. We wanted to be finished with that stage of life, to stop worrying about it. The diaphragm had failed us twice. Belinda had side effects from the pill. We simply couldn't see putting 24 dozen pills of any kind into her system each year for another twenty years. Three friends had become pregnant on the IUD; and condoms, jellies, withdrawal, and abstinence were all unacceptable to us for reasons of questionable effectiveness or aesthetic-sexual distaste. We also wanted to avoid the trauma of abortion. Sterilization was

the only means which was 100 per cent reliable (99 per cent was n◄
enough for us) which did not depend on some messy, awkward,
and distasteful artificial device, and which was perfectly safe
and healthy.

The key reason we decided on a vasectomy rather than
tubal ligation was that the hoary Sterilization/Abortion Committee at New York Hospital had the effrontery not to permit
Belinda to be sterilized because she was too young (she'd only
been voting for 8 years!) and because she had too few children
(only 3!). Only our utter amazement and absolute incredulity
at this outrageous imposition of policy (an outmoded one at
that) and invasion of personal rights of adult parents prevented
our bringing a lawsuit against the hospital. What right has a
committee of doctors or anyone else to concern itself with,
much less make a decision about, our personal family size?

After our initial shock, we learned that another hospital
and doctor in New York would accommodate us. By that time,
however, we had begun to consider a vasectomy. After much
investigation and soul searching, we realized that it was more
logical — cheaper, quicker, less painful, less of an operation,
and equally effective.

Since we felt quite alone in our decision, we benefited
greatly from the experience, assistance, and enthusiasm of the
Association for Voluntary Sterilization. They sent us brochures,
news clippings, and medical opinions — and the name of a
cooperating urologist. Belinda and I met him, as per his request, to discuss the significance and technical details of a
vasectomy. Then we both signed a statement to the effect we
understood I would no longer be able to father any children.
The doctor examined me briefly and we decided on "V" day.

When the hour finally came at the end of work one day
a week later, I braced myself on the way to the doctor's office
with the contents of two mini-bottles of Scotch. After a local
anesthetic, which hurt more than anything that followed, I
was somewhat surprised at the lack of pain. The major discomfort during the 15-minute operation was the anxiety and
expectation of pain. Half an hour after my arrival, I was on my
way home, walking carefully and looking like a sore cowboy.

The next day I rested at home with considerable awareness of local soreness. The day after that, I returned to work quite pleased and smug. The bruised feeling lasted for some weeks but gradually disappeared; the minor swelling went down within ten days; the ¼-inch scars and internal stitching were no longer noticeable after a year.

Within a week of the operation, my determination to demonstrate that I hadn't lost anything important overcame my fear of hurting what I had left. Though somewhat restrained, we were reassured that I could still perform sexually to our satisfaction. A week later the sperm count in the doctor's office indicated we were "home free" — I was perfectly sterile, though not the least bit less virile.

What a joyful combination! For the two years since then we have been utterly free from worry about pregnancy and absolutely unconcerned about contraceptive devices. Making love is the spontaneous expressive event it should be, as it now has nothing to do with making babies. (This may be part of the reason that obstetricians and hospital committees are reluctant to promote sterilization — they fear lost customers!)

My wife claims I am more masculine than before the operation. I think I have gained a fuller confidence in knowing that my claim to manhood lies in personal characteristics other than my sperm count. If for whatever reasons I may have become a better husband, I know I have gained more in my wife. She has proof I no longer want her as a baby machine — I want and need more than that in a life partner. As a result, she has been able to plan her life without the fear that it will be interrupted again by a pregnancy and baby raising. She is now able to resume her career as a teacher, which in turn has made her a happier person, a more confidant and capable mother, and a more responsive and interesting wife. Viva la vasectomy!

A postscript on questions often asked: 1) No, there is no change in your sex life. The only difference may be an increased frequency as making love is easier, more spontaneous, uninhibited and natural — without the paraphernalia or fear. 2) Yes, we did consider the possibilities of divorce, death, and

change of mind. We felt we couldn't plan our life in expectation of tragedy, that everyone makes irreversible decisions in
many areas. Children are not like pets, to be replaced if they
are run over. And to us the possibility of another pregnancy
was a worse prospect than the possibility of changing our minds
about having more children. 3) Yes, Women's Lib will catch on
to vasectomies. Except for the problem of the overblown male
ego, vasectomy is much more sensible than female sterilization. And it is about time that man learned that it is not his
sperm count but his willingness and ability to please his woman
that matters. 4) No, I don't think vasectomy is the answer for
every male, but I am firmly convinced that a level-headed
appraisal will show every couple, secure in its marriage and
complete in its childbearing, that sterilization is the easiest
and most sensible method of permanent contraception. No one
wants an unexpected baby, but anyone using other forms of
birth control is asking for it. Whether the couple chooses
male or female sterilization is much less important — what
matters is that a single act can take care of all your birth
control problems for the rest of your active life.

6 AT 22, MY HUSBAND CHOSE STERILIZATION

Anonymous, as told to Fredelle Maynard

When I tell anyone that my husband had a *vasectomy,*
the usual reaction is, "At *his* age?" People are getting accustomed to the idea that at 45 or 50, say, a man might choose
to be sterilized. But Terry is only 22. Even close friends seem
to think there's something strange about a young man decid-
ing he's not going to father any more children. "I didn't know
you took the population explosion so seriously," somebody
said to me. The answer is I do — we do — take very seriously
the population explosion on our own doorstep. Yes, I'm concerned about all those grim scientific predictions of what will
happen to our world if the birth rate isn't checked. But I don't
think we'd have been personally moved to take action if we

hadn't found ourselves, after four years of marriage, with three children — and the prospect of a fertile quarter-century ahead.

I met Terry over a Bunsen burner in high school chemistry lab and — well, he really lit a flame right off. Neither of us dated anybody else after that. By our senior year we were talking marriage. Not right away, of course. Terry would go to college and study hotel administration. I planned secretarial training. And as soon as we had a little money saved, we'd settle down and start raising a family. Two boys and two girls, a pleasant house not too far from the city, a dog and a flower garden. . . . I had it all worked out.

Except that the summer after graduation we both realized we wanted to be together all the time. My parents agreed to let us rent three rooms in their house, and we were married on my eighteenth birthday. I really didn't mind not having a place of my own right off. Anyway, it would be only for a little while, until we could afford an apartment. Terry took a job as stock clerk in an automotive supply store; I got work as a doctor's receptionist. Between the two of us, we were earning close to $800 a month. We bought a rug, made a down payment on a stove and refrigerator and began to talk about turning in our jalopy for a new car.

Naturally we didn't plan on babies for quite some time. I don't recall, though, that we ever discussed contraception. I just assumed Terry would take care of things, and Terry assumed we'd rely on the one kind of birth control he knew anything about — male condoms. But both of us disliked using them. He began to take chances. Sometimes — when we figured it was my "safe period" — he didn't take any precautions at all. So I guess we shouldn't have been surprised when, two months after the wedding, I found I was pregnant.

At first I was terribly upset. Pregnancy meant giving up my job — with those furniture payments still to meet — and staying on in my parents' house. Where would we even put a baby? But Terry was reassuring. He almost persuaded me it would be an advantage, having the first child when we were so young. I worked another two months, until it became clear that I wasn't going to have one of those dream pregnancies where everything goes exactly right. I had an unusually long period of morning sickness, then backache, swelling of the ankles and — almost from the start — an overwhelming fatigue. So I threw in the sponge, and Terry — claiming it was no hardship, he *liked* being busy — took a second job as a security guard. Cheryl was born while her daddy was on night duty. I remember feeling disappointed that I'd missed the traditional new-mother moment, my husband kneeling by the bedside and murmuring, "Darling, you were wonderful! We have a beautiful baby."

Cheryl *was* beautiful and good, but her arrival changed our lives in ways I couldn't have imagined. Until then, we'd kept something of the high school courtship pattern going — out to dinner occasionally, driving the 40 miles to New York for a show, dancing, flowers for no reason and sentimental presents. Now we had to watch every penny; baby expenses came to well over $1,000.

Even if we'd had extra money, we were both too tired to be interested in night life. "A great night for me," Terry said once, "would be eight hours of sleep." When I went for my six-week checkup the obstetrician said, "You're pushing yourself pretty hard, aren't you? I'd advise putting off the next pregnancy for at least two years." I left his office with a diaphragm and the determination that this time we'd be careful about birth control.

The trouble with the diaphragm was that it spoiled something I'd always valued in our sex life — its spontaneity. Using a diaphragm means being prepared in advance; it's an awful nuisance if you just feel suddenly and happily amorous.

For the first time in our married life we began to bicker about sex. Terry claimed I was always putting him off. I said it was all very well for *him* to be casual; he couldn't get pregnant and he wouldn't have to look after *two* babies. Inevitably, one night I gave in when he told me *coitus interruptus* was perfectly safe: he would withdraw before ejaculation, and there'd be no possibility of conception. We tried it — and then came Cathy.

That next year, with the four of us living in three rooms, was a nightmare. Cathy was a difficult baby from the start. She came home from the hospital with an infected navel. She had terrible colic; would wake screaming with pain; we took turns rocking her so the noise wouldn't disturb my parents. Then she had a series of costly allergy tests before we discovered she couldn't take cow's milk (after which she graduated to soybean milk at 50 cents a can). We spent so much time in the doctor's office that he joked about giving us a monthly rate.

Meantime, I had gone on the Pill and was having a bad time with it. At least, I blamed my depression on the Pill, but maybe that's unfair. Certainly I had plenty to be depressed about. Looking after two babies — Cheryl was 18 months old when Cathy was born — took all my strength. Though Terry was still moonlighting, the extra money scarcely kept up with the bills. We had no privacy. My parents did their best to be understanding, but it was clear that when they first offered to share their house, they'd been thinking of two people, not four.

I don't know who was most upset when I became pregnant a third time. Terry was angry ("I thought you were taking care!"). I was reproachful, reminding him about the times he'd talked me into taking a chance after I'd forgotten my Pill. And my mother was frantic: "You'll be worn out before you're thirty!"

I must say that sometimes, after Andrea was born, I did feel a hundred years old. We'd moved to an apartment — small, but more than we could afford. Terry and I were both working too hard; we quarreled over little things, or nothing. As for our sex life — I'd gone back to using a diaphragm, but was constantly nervous that something might go wrong. It got so I tensed up whenever Terry touched me. I knew our marriage couldn't stand the strain of another "accident."

The idea of permanent birth control first occurred to me when a friend had her tubes tied after a fourth, unplanned baby. The gynecologist I consulted wasn't too encouraging, though. Yes, *salpingectomy* (the cutting or tying of the female

Fallopian tubes) was legal in almost all states, and he was quite willing to perform it. But individual hospitals established their own policy in this matter, and the hospital in our small city, he was sure, would not approve my being sterilized ("You're so young"). I could have the operation performed elsewhere, no doubt, but that would involve travel and additional expense. Out of sheer disappointment and frustration I burst into tears. The doctor patted my hand. "My dear, I'm sure if you *do* have more babies, you'll love them just the same." *That isn't the point,* I thought. *We already have as many children as we want, and can properly provide for.*

That night we experienced the most serious crisis of our marriage. Just before bedtime, I began to feel faint. Lying down made the dizziness worse. Suddenly I was suffocating. The more I gasped, the harder it became to breathe. By the time Terry got me to the hospital, I was scarcely conscious. There, the doctor who examined me said the attack was purely nervous in origin. Physically I was fine, but I must see a psychiatrist as soon as possible. That scared me so much I got as far as making an appointment. Thinking about it, though, I became convinced it wasn't a psychiatrist I needed. What I needed was rest; the chance to spend some quiet time alone with my husband, and freedom from the constant fear of an unwanted pregnancy. I'd heard about vasectomy — not from my doctor, oddly enough, but from a magazine article. I wrote to the Association for Voluntary Sterilization and got a list of physicians in our area who performed this simple operation.

Terry was hesitant to begin with. Naturally, he wanted to be absolutely sure that vasectomy wouldn't affect his sexual performance or satisfaction. On that point the doctor put our minds at rest. Vasectomy is not castration; it involves no glands or organs. It merely prevents impregnation by closing off the two small tubes that carry sperm from the testicles. The male sex hormone is not affected; the body continues to produce (and absorb) sperm. Everything happens exactly as before — except that the semen contains no sperm. And the simple procedure — two small incisions in the scrotum, so the tubes (vas deferens) can be cut and tied — could be performed

in the doctor's office under a local anesthetic. Terry needn't
even miss a day's work.

On the doctor's advice, we took a month to think things
over before signing the consent form that authorized Terry's
vasectomy. During that time we discussed, very seriously, the
questions raised during our joint interview. What if, in five or
ten years, we decided we wanted another child? (Sometimes,
after vasectomy, the tubes can be untied and rejoined. But
there's no guarantee that the original operation is reversible.) Terry and I felt the same way: If we ever wanted to increase our family, we'd adopt. The world is full of homeless
children. I think I'd be inclined to choose an Indian child,
maybe, or a child of mixed racial heritage — the kind of young-
ster agencies find hard to place. And I'd take a four- or five-
year-old, not a baby. Some women, I know, really enjoy the
utter dependency of infancy; the baby's helplessness makes
them feel loved and necessary. I'm not at my best with in-
fants. I feel loved and necessary when I'm reading to Cheryl
and Cathy, dancing with them to records, taking them to the
zoo and showing them how to bake cookies. Once I get Andrea
into training pants, I'll be ready to turn my back on the diaper-
changing, bottle-heating routines.

Another question the doctor asked: "Have you considered how you'd feel if, after a vasectomy, your three children were lost in some tragic accident?" I didn't have to think
long about that. If such a catastrophe occurred, my problem
would be to pull myself together and go on. How could I think
of "replacing" my three little girls? And what if — unthinkable
as it seems now — Terry and I divorced and he were to marry
again? Well, he'd still be the father of three children, responsible for them. That's quite a lot, in the modern world.

If our financial situation were to improve enormously,
would we then regret being unable to produce more children?
I can honestly say NO. True, right now our budget is one of the
things that makes reliable contraception necessary. But even
if we had plenty of money, I wouldn't wish to bear another
child. I can see now that the old dream of two boys and two
girls is not for me. Much as I enjoy my children, I don't want

to go on for the next ten years washing hands and getting drinks of water. I have obligations to myself and to my husband. I want Terry to have a chance at that hotel training he's always longed for. I want, when the girls are in school, to do something on my own, maybe run a small business. I'd like us to be free to travel. In short, I'm already thinking of my long-range future with Terry — of us not simply as parents, but as lovers, co-workers, *friends*.

Oh, sure, I can believe that in ten years I might see a new mother cuddling her baby and think, "Wouldn't it be nice if . . . ?" But in ten years Cheryl will be 14, even Andrea will be a big girl. That's late to introduce another baby into a household, imposing on the older children part of the work and responsibility a baby brings. And 20 years from now . . . well, I'll still be of childbearing age, but by that time I'll be looking forward to becoming a *grandmother*.

Are there any disadvantages to a vasectomy? Perhaps it wouldn't be suitable for a man unsure of his masculinity. But for us it seems ideal. It was inexpensive — $175 — and in no way disabling. It's sure. As for its effect on our sexual relationship — something I know people are curious about, though they hesitate to ask — it's been truly liberating. Our lovemaking is free from anxiety and fear. And now, with the assurance that our family is complete, we can make confident plans for the future.

7 A FEMINIST CASE FOR VASECTOMY

by Anselma Dell 'Olio

A charter member of the National Organization for Women, Anselma Dell 'Olio is founder and director of the New Feminist Theater, and a commentator on radio station WRFM, New York.

This paper is based on a feminist premise — that women have been and are severely discriminated against in political, economic, and social spheres, a situation morally intolerable; that the perpetrators of discrimination are not an anonymous "they"; and that such discrimination has proven to be solely for the advantage of men. They and only they are responsible for the inequality so destructive of human potential and the ability to achieve happiness.

The attempts by antifeminists to place the burden of oppression on the oppressed (i.e., "women are their own worst enemies") is a falsehood frequently employed by those in power who cannot or will not face up to their responsibility and ensuing guilt for having been, wittingly or unwittingly, the agents of oppression.

A tenet basic to radical feminism (not to be confused with the organization known as the Radical Feminists) is that the nuclear family serves no useful or healthy purpose, and is in fact an intrinsic part of the fabric of female oppression. The radical feminist philosophy maintains that the nuclear family must be eliminated as a prerequisite of female emancipation, along with the automatic ownership of children by biological or adoptive "parents." We can only conjecture about the reasons why women are subjugated to men. What is clear is that the discovery of paternity played and continues to play an important role in this subjugation. Because of this, ownership and lines of heredity were established; the false link between a man's virility and fertility was able to develop into a philosophy we might call the "masculine mystique." The idea that there is some divine connection between sperm and the metaphysical quality of "manhood" or virility, in itself a sophistry, has reached cult and totem proportions in our (patriarchal) society. Even men of intelligence and ability like Norman Mailer can maintain doggedly and in the face of contrary evidence that such a link not only exists, but is crucial to the well-being of humanity (cf. "Prisoner of Sex").

Thus the ultimate goal of radical feminists must be to revert to a state where paternity (and through technology, perhaps maternity) become irrelevant. Further, because political subjugation of women was largely made possible by their biological subjugation, which condemned them to chain pregnancies; weakened, debilitated, and doomed them to short lives of pain and discomfort, it becomes obvious that only through

absolute control over reproduction could women reaffirm
their humanity and shake off the bonds of male dominance.

Temporary methods of birth control, as they exist today,
are all too obviously inadequate. Drastic measures are called
for not just to eliminate female oppression, but to salvage
humanity from reproducing itself beyond the capacity of the
environment to sustain its numbers which daily increase through
geometrical progression at a dizzying speed. The only clear
answer that technology has to offer is male sterilization. It
is easy, fast, safe, efficient, and cheap. It involves a minimum
of discomfort and time, and psychological problems have proved
almost nonexistent in motivated males.

Naturally, there is no greater threat to the "masculine
mystique" than to advocate vasectomy. However, men who
mean business about Women's Liberation are going to have to
face up to their responsibilities and take the initiative in the
prevention of unwanted pregnancies. With the exception of the
very primitive condom and error-prone coitus interruptus, men
have never assumed such responsibility. After all, they rarely
pay the price, if ever, in human terms, and need never pay in
material terms if they do not wish to.

Supposedly women want children more than men. And
men often complain of having been made "family men" in-
voluntarily. Yet women, brainwashed as they are ("programmed"
or "conditioned" might be better words), and hog-tied from
operating in a free context, of course *use* their sexuality (including reproductive capacity) to bargain for what they want.
And having babies (i.e., "getting knocked up") is one of the
age-old methods — one of the few available to them — for
making themselves more valuable to (i.e., "trap") a man.

If a man she loves has a vasectomy, a woman will perhaps be forced to take those first (or even second) steps towards
her own liberation. Such ingrained values as motherhood die
hard. But if she falls in love with a man who is or becomes
willfully sterile, she may actually be forced to liberate herself from defining her validity as a human being solely as a
childbearer and rearer. In this context, vasectomy can be a
revolutionary and feminist action for a man — a demonstration

of sincere love and support and positive affirmation. What could be more humanly beneficial than to hear a man say or declare by his actions that he loves a woman not because of her capacity to bear *his* biological offspring, but because she is a human being whom he desires and respects and wants (not *needs*) to be with and make love to for her own intrinsic value?

REFERENCES:

Simone de Beauvoir, *The Second Sex* (New York: Modern Library, 1968)
Caroline Bird with Sara Welles Briller, *Born Female* (New York: David McKay, 1968)
Shulamith Firestone, *The Dialectic of Sex* (New York: William Morrow, 1970)
Germaine Greer, *The Female Eunuch* (New York: McGraw-Hill, 1971)
Kate Millet, *Sexual Politics* (Garden City, N.Y.: Doubleday, 1970)

8 STERILIZATION

Talk presented to New York County Medical Society, May 11, 1970

by Helen Edey, M.D.

I believe that sterilization is a method of family planning which should be considered rationally on its merits when it might be indicated, and this is not always done. In my view, it should be thoroughly considered whenever a person is *sure* that he or she never wants any more children. The reasons for this decision are various, and of course may include medical reasons such as chronic illness, physical or mental, inheritable diseases, poor health of the mother due to multiparity, and economic reasons. But a very common reason is that a couple simply wishes to lead a kind of life which does not include the care of more young children, and that is a perfectly valid reason.

So why not contraception? The person who wishes sterilization has four main objections to contraception. First, the failure rates are too high. Use effectiveness is of course quite different from theoretical effectiveness, and it is widely known that mechanical methods are not thoroughly reliable, partly because they must be used at the time of coitus and are, therefore, subject to the temporary feelings and impulses of either partner, or the perhaps unfavorable environment of the moment. The Population Council states that, for the diaphragm in the United States, "in clinical practice, a pregnancy rate of 10 per 100 women per year is quite satisfactory." Over a period of 15 years, it has been estimated that a person using a mechanical method has a 50% chance or more of having another child. The IUD may, of course, be expelled or require removal in up to 20% of cases, but even if successfully retained, Dr. Tietze of the Population Council tells me that the risk of pregnancy is about 15% in 10 years. The pill is subject to forgetting due to simple misunderstanding, or to a syndrome which Dr. Hans Lehfeldt has called "Willful Exposure to Unwanted Pregnancy," and which involves many psychological conflicts. Many people are unwilling to take all the above chances.

A second objection to contraception is, of course, the occurrence of side-effects which we have already heard a good deal about in the U.S. recently. A third is the simple objection to having to insert, remember, or be esthetically bothered by various methods. The fourth objection is one which I believe is under-estimated: chronic fears, either of pregnancy which preoccupies many couples monthly and often with each act of intercourse and which can affect sexual relations and general contentment, or exaggerated fears of the side-effects of the pill.

With these indications, and the large number of people who want no more children, why isn't sterilization even more common? One reason that there are not more here is that there is a great deal of ignorance about sterilization; laymen may hardly have heard of vasectomy, though they generally know of "tying the tubes," but unfortunately many doctors also have misconceptions. There are certainly psychological blocks to considering this procedure, especially in the male. Men confuse sterilization with castration, and even if reassured, many cannot resolve this anxiety. I believe that male doctors are not im-

mune to this problem. In historical times, sterilization has
been used in a punitive way, and included castration to induce
docility. In some countries it is still considered mutilation.
Some doctors still believe that sterilization here, especially
vasectomy, is illegal, and I find that quite mysterious when so
many tubal ligations are done openly in hospitals. Actually,
voluntary sterilization is legal in every state for any indication
at all, except in Utah and Connecticut, where medical necessity
is required, and that requirement has just been repealed in
Connecticut effective in [October] 1971. Doctors maintain
that they are afraid of lawsuits, though the fact is that none
has ever been won against a doctor when proper consent has
been signed, and very few are even threatened. As a psychiatrist,
I suspect some rationalization here. There are many administrative obstacles to tubal ligations in hospitals where various
formulae are adopted which, to my mind, are irrelevant to a
rational evaluation of a particular case.

Vasectomy is quicker, safer and cheaper than tubal
ligation, does not involve getting a hospital bed or the approval
of a committee, and so if the husband wishes, it may be the
preferred procedure. It involves a 20-minute operation generally
using local anesthesia. Incisions are made over each mobilized
vas deferens. The sheath of the vas is opened, and the vas is
brought out through the scrotum. It is doubly clamped and
cut. A segment from 1-3 cm. is removed, for confirmation by
a pathologist. Each end is then tied with a non-absorbable
suture. Some urologists also coagulate the lumen. The sheath
should then be closed over each end, and the scrotum closed
with absorbable sutures. There may be local discomfort and
swelling for several days, but most men can return to work in a
day or two. There is no interference with hormone production
nor with the secretions ejaculated, so that sexual desire and
intercourse, including ejaculation, are unchanged. After the
operation, about ten ejaculations are usually needed to dispose
of the store of sperm cells; the patient must be required to return for semen analyses until the laboratory has reported
azospermia, and until then contraception must be used.

With the fear of pregnancy removed, sexual activity is

often more enjoyable. In a review of 23 papers reporting results of vasectomy, the degree of almost complete satisfaction averages over 95%. The latest and largest study is a report of over 1,000 cases by the Simon Population Trust in England in 1969. In their series, the patient's sexual life improved 73.1%, remained the same in 25.4% and deteriorated in 1.5%.

The rate of spontaneous reanastomosis is presently under one-half of one percent and declining with improved techniques. The patient should be asked to return for semen analysis after one year to check on this rare possibility. Surgical reversibility has been attained in various degrees by different investigators, from 50% to 80%. However, it has been found that in many men after vasectomy, an apparent antigen-antibody reaction has developed, and even after surgical reanastomosis there may be azospermia, or the spermatozoa may have a high percent of head-tail separation and are not sufficiently viable to cause pregnancy. This phenomenon will be a problem with any of the supposedly reversible techniques which are under study or being proposed, such as plugs, clips or intra-vas devices, and the operation must be considered irreversible at this time. However, there is still a very large number of men, and I mean in the millions in the U.S. alone, who might be candidates for vasectomy and who have no interest in reversibility. Requests for reversal now run around 1% in men.

To turn now to female sterilization, male doctors have been a little less reluctant to perform tubal ligations, but still have hedged themselves around with administrative committees and regulations. Even the most liberal hospitals will use the so-called parity formula: age times number of children equals 120, though the most recent American College of Obstetrics and Gynecology guidelines explicitly state that this is not necessary. In New York, Puerto Rican women commonly go to Puerto Rico for a sterilization after being refused here. (In 1965, it was estimated that one-third of all Puerto Rican women between 20 and 49 years had been sterilized.) Some hysterectomies for minimal uterine pathology are really for sterilization purposes and are done to get around these rules.

The operation is most conveniently done post-partum; at that time it is technically easier, and there is high motivation, but there is a higher failure rate, being one in 200 with the Pomeroy procedure, double the usual one. One sub-umbilical incision is made, and the uterus is deflected first to one side and then the other. Several other techniques may be used for an internal sterilization. In the vaginal approach, either the anterior or posterior cul-de-sac may be entered, with or without a culdoscope. In the Irving technique, an abdominal one, the proximal segment of the tube is turned and buried in the myometrium, resulting in a very low failure rate, but it takes longer.

In order to minimize hospital stay and develop a possible outpatient procedure, many new techniques are being studied. The laparoscope is being used in several centers to penetrate the abdominal wall. A special electrical instrument is inserted which first coagulates and then cuts the tubes. This process takes 20 minutes; there is no scar, no ileus, and the patient may leave in 12 hours or so.

The transcervical route is being used to introduce caustics. Zipper in Chile has been using quinacrine for this purpose, with an obstruction rate of 84% after two instillations. The electrocautery is favored by some experimenters, but regarded as unsafe by others. Freezing of the uterine cornus with liquid nitrogen or freon is being tried, with a claimed success rate of 80%. Temporary occlusion of the fallopian tube has been attempted by the injection of a liquid silicone polymer that vulcanizes at body temperature to form a plug, but these appear to be readily dislodged.

Attempts at reversibility have resulted in an average pregnancy rate of about 25%. Before trying this procedure, both spouses should have a fertility work-up, and the woman a pre-operative hysterogram. There has been one request for reversal in about 1,000 sterilizations.

Who should be considered for sterilization? I am presently engaged in screening the applicants for vasectomy at the new Vasectomy Service at the Margaret Sanger Research Bureau, which opened here October 1, [1969]. New Yorkers may be interested to know that we have been swamped with applications from all over the country, having received over 1,000 inquiries in March alone. A large percentage of these applicants have been refused vasectomy by private urologists. I conduct about an hour's interview with the couple, which includes a discussion of the possibilities of death of the children, or of the spouse and remarriage. I ask about, and try to evaluate, any anxieties either member of the couple may have about the effects of the operation. I look for signs of pressure by one spouse on the other; both must want it sincerely or there may be later regrets and resentment; I try also to estimate the stability of the relationship. Feelings about possible adoption are explored. Any magical expectation of a cure for sexual problems or marital discord would be a contra-indication, as would be irrational fears of loss of masculinity.

I find about 90% of the applicants who come to an interview to be mature men in their thirties and forties for whom I think vasectomy is the procedure of choice. Considering the population problem we have all been talking about, I think that sterilization can serve a more prominent role than it has in the past.

9　VASECTOMY: HOW TO MEET AND SURVIVE A WAVE OF DEMAND

by Curtis Wood, Jr., M.D.

Partly because of the efforts of the Association for Voluntary Sterilization, whose speakers now reach some 20 million Americans a year through radio and television programs, and also because of the great increase in space given to the subject by the lay press and news media, more married couples have become aware of sterilization as a method of controlling the size of their families, and the public has come to understand just what sterilization is and is not.

It is quite possible that the women's liberation movement has played an important role in the increased popularity of vasectomy. Traditionally, if a man's wife — or girl friend — became unwillingly pregnant, the man would become indignant and accuse her of being stupid because she had not taken suitable precautions. Seldom was it his fault.

Except for withdrawal and the condom, methods of contraception have involved the woman — douches, jellies, creams, suppositories, diaphragms, IUDs, The Pill, and rhythm. But now, women have heard about vasectomy, and we can imagine one saying: "Why should I bother taking a pill, which might be harmful, twenty days of every month and twelve months of every year for twenty more years and thus enable you to have the sexual relations you want without the babies you do not want? I think you should have a vasectomy instead and relieve me of this burden."

It is probably true that imagined or actual sexual capacities are more intimately related to the male's ego than they are to the woman's. It is partly for this reason that some men are reluctant to terminate their fertility. If a man really feels — and this is more an emotional than an intellectual reaction — that being unable to impregnate a woman is a reflection on his masculinity, then he should not have a vasectomy. A Milquetoast who may possibly be pressured, by a domineering wife or a meddling mother-in-law, to have this operation that he really fears and dreads is quite apt to develop undesirable psychological side effects. These are the possible 1 or 2 percent of men who have regretted their vasectomies, according to several surveys. It has been shown that many of this small minority had psychiatric problems prior to the vasectomy, but adequate preoperative interviewing should screen out most of them.

OPENING UP

Only a few years ago, people were hesitant to discuss contraceptive techniques, abortion, and sterilization on a personal basis. Many women did not want it known that they were on The Pill, and men kept their vasectomies as secret as possible. But times have changed, and we more easily discuss these matters with friends or in public, and sterilizations — of both men and women — have become more socially acceptable.

Men such as Arthur Godfrey and Paul Ehrlich have frequently said on radio and TV programs that they have had this operation, and they recommend it highly for those who are sure they will never want more children.

SEX-STATUS SYMBOL

A recent issue of *The New York Times* contained an article on sterilization, in which three men and three women who had been sterilized gave their reasons for this choice. They even permitted their pictures to be used. The Association for Voluntary Sterilization has designed a gold lapel-pin, consisting of the male sex symbol with a small section removed, to be worn as a kind of status symbol by members of the club. In a few months' time, over 3,000 pins were sold, and they are now working on a pin for women who have been demanding a similar marker.

In the past, many hospitals had sterilization committees that had to approve of every tubal ligation, and many of these committees had strict requirements, such as a genuine medical indication or a certain number of children for specific age groups. These committee attitudes were often based on suggestions — not requirements — of the American College of Obstetricians and Gynecologists, as expressed in their *Manual of Standards*. The 1969 edition, however, deleted entirely the age-parity section and said: "Many states have no statutes on sterilization. In the latter it can be performed on anyone who is legally capable of giving consent for the operation. Regardless of state laws, however, each hospital must establish its own regulations concerning sterilization. . . . Since there are important emotional problems relating to sterilization, it is essential that consultation be obtained before the operation is performed. In a few hospitals committee review, like that for therapeutic abortion, is required; but in most the permission of two senior obstetricians is all that is necessary."

This suggestion from the ACOG indicates that committee action on sterilizations is no longer indicated nor necessary, and it may explain why more and more hospitals are dropping the sterilization committee. In a large San Diego hospital, the obstetrical resident may be the single required consultant.

"IDEAL CONTRACEPTIVE"

The majority of vasectomies are performed in the doctor's office. This avoids the problems caused by hospital regulations. Apparently, some physicians still believe that the AMA does not approve of vasectomies; they must have missed the editorial in the issue of *JAMA,* May 27, 1968, which states: "Voluntary sterilization of man is safe, quick, effective and legal. Yet physicians are reluctant to use the procedure even though it seems to offer the ideal contraceptive for a husband when his family has become as large as he and his wife want or can afford. Why do these men, particularly if they are in the lower income... population, have so much difficulty obtaining a sterilization operation?"

The editorial then discusses these reasons and shows most of them are not valid.

To help remedy the situation that the *JAMA* editorial deplored, an outpatient vasectomy clinic was opened in New York City in the fall of 1969. Since then, in only a little over a year, similar clinics have been established all over the United States. They have all had two major problems in common: finding physicians to staff the clinic; and determining how to avoid a long waiting list of patients. As of December 1971, there were about 175 outpatient vasectomy clinics in the U.S.

Some urologists fear that if it became known that they do office vasectomies they would be swamped with requests. This has been a common experience, and it is understandable that these highly trained and skillful surgeons would shudder at the thought of doing vasectomies all day long on an assembly-line basis. For them, there is little that is stimulating or challenging about a vasectomy. But if the physician realizes the absolute necessity of stopping the population increase; if he acknowledges that it is people who pollute, and the more people the more pollution; if he wants to preserve some quality of life for his children and grandchildren; and if he appreciates that, in most cases, marriages are improved for both hus-

band and wife by this procedure, then he can have a sense of reward that could offset the boredom of vasectomies. We physicians
are also citizens of this country; we cannot concentrate just on
medicine and leave all else to the social workers, economists,
politicians, and lawyers.

It is possible to control the situation by each week setting
aside a certain period during which a given number of operations will be done. If more urologists were willing to help
meet the demand for this medical service, those who are
trying to cooperate would not have such long waiting lists.
Some urologists are apparently finding vasectomies sufficiently
profitable and stimulating to make this a kind of subspecialty.
One physician in California recently reported to the Association for Voluntary Sterilization that he had just done his 10,000th
vasectomy, and there are others who average 250 a year.

What does all this portend? Well, looking into the
crystal ball is both fascinating and dangerous, but perhaps we
can make a few predictions anyway.

The young people of America are extremely concerned
about the deterioration of our environment. The phenomenal
growth of the Zero Population Growth organization — mostly
through college chapters — shows that these future parents
are willing to stop at two children of their own and adopt
however many more may be wanted. The group has grown
from 100 members to 25,000 in about a year and a half.

As all forms of pollution increase, as the environment
continues to deteriorate (it inevitably will for years to come),
and as the staggering $10 billion welfare bill — so much of
which goes for aid to dependent (and frequently unwanted)
children — continues to soar, families with more than two
children will go out of style and be increasingly condemned,
socially. An effective, long-term contraceptive method will
become more and more in demand.

Even if the present restrictive abortion laws in most
states are repealed; if the prostaglandins prove to be the
simple, safe, cheap, sure-fire abortion-pill; and even if these
are available in slot machines everywhere, still, prevention of
a pregnancy will always be preferable to terminating it.

Therefore, I predict that in the foreseeable future the demand for vasectomy will continue, will grow, and more urologists as well as general practitioners and osteopathic physicians will have to become involved in meeting that demand. Although new methods of fertility control will be developed in the next few years, sterilization will remain the method of choice for many couples when family size is complete.

Part Two ♀♂

Making the Decision

1 MALE OR FEMALE STERILIZATION?

by Donald J. Dodds, M.D.

It is a great deal easier to sterilize a man than a woman.
The operation on a man can be done in a doctor's office or in
the outpatient department of a hospital. A local anaesthetic
(popularly called "freezing") is normally used. The operation
is done through one or two small incisions in the scrotum,
the pouch that holds the testicles. There is little discomfort
and the man can ordinarily return to work in a day or two. In
contrast, the operation on a woman has to be done in hospital.
There is more discomfort and a longer period of convalescence.
Because the vaginal method is relatively new it is not available
at all medical centres, and in addition, is not suitable for all
women.

It would appear that because the operation on a man is
simpler, it would be the first choice. In general this is true, and
certainly is so from a purely surgical point of view. But other
factors must be taken into consideration. Each couple must
consider all aspects of the matter, and should consult with their
family physician, or other respected advisor, if they are in
doubt.

ATTITUDES TOWARDS STERILIZATION

No one should attempt to talk a man into having a sterilization operation. It must be a free choice based on his conviction that this is something he wants to do for his own benefit and for the benefit of others involved.

A not insignificant proportion of the male population are firmly convinced that if they were rendered incapable of making women pregnant they would no longer be men. This attitude may be due to lack of knowledge of the facts. If so, providing the correct information may enable such a man, in time, to change his point of view, and become a suitable subject for sterilization. But if he is not only firmly convinced but also emotionally bound to this attitude, no amount of reasoning will change his conviction. Persuading such a man to undergo a sterilization operation could lead to him suffering from feelings of inadequacy.

Such a fear is to be distinguished from every man's need to be reassured that the operation will not interfere with his normal enjoyment of sexual intercourse. The man who wishes to make certain of this before proceeding with the operation is exercising his intelligence and the natural instinct to protect his completeness. From Nature's point of view he stands to lose something — the ability to reproduce. But from a human point of view he stands to gain something — the greater ability to control his life.

Some women are convinced that sterilization would cause them a loss of femininity, and, as with the men, sterilization in such instances would not be in their best interests.

WHEN STERILIZATION IS CALLED FOR

Sterilization of men or women is indicated whenever they no longer wish to produce children. However, this is not a decision to be made lightly, nor should the operation be performed immediately after the decision is made. Most people who have been sterilized express satisfaction with the results and continue to be satisfied throughout the rest of their lives. Because it brings relief from the fear of unwanted pregnancies, there is often more enjoyment of intercourse, more confidence in planning for the future, and generally better relations between husband and wife. Occasionally there are incidents of dissatisfaction and regret, but most of these could be avoided if attention were paid to the considerations discussed in the following paragraphs.

PREPARING TO MAKE THE DECISION

Before a man is sterilized he and his wife should feel comfortable with the idea, and should think over and thoroughly discuss the following questions:

1.   Is either of us afraid that the operation might change our feelings about ourselves, about each other, or about how other people regard us?

It is natural to feel some apprehension about an operation. But before a vasectomy is performed, a man should thoroughly discuss and resolve his anxieties, if any, about how sterilization might alter his regard for himself and for his wife, his wife's feelings towards him and other people's evaluation of his decision and subsequent condition. Similarly, a wife should examine her feelings about herself, her husband and others. They should both feel comfortable with the idea that they will no longer have the potential ability to share in the creation of new life; the man will not be able to cause a pregnancy, nor will his wife be able to be made pregnant by him.

2.   Are we likely to regret that we cannot have more children?

When they first marry, many people feel that they would like to have a moderately large family, but later often modify their ideas when they discover the many emotional, social and financial problems associated with raising children. Some of these problems, such as financial difficulties, may be only temporary, and when they subside the desire for more children may return. This desire is sometimes satisfied by adopting children, but adoption has certain associated problems, and does not give exactly the same satisfactions that come from having one's own children.

3. Do we both completely agree on the operation being done?

Lack of complete agreement between husband and wife appears to be the most common cause of emotional problems following sterilization. This may take several forms. A man may feel he is being pressured by his wife, his relatives, his doctor or his wife's doctor, into having the operation; or by circumstances — financial, social or health. Sterilization may be the best solution to the existing problems, but because he has not fully accepted it a man may carry a resentment for the rest of his life. A wife whose husband decides to have the operation without consulting her, and then gets her to sign a consent agreement by belittling and scorning her anxieties, is likely to harbour resentment and anxiety about his motives which will come between them. Two people who hurriedly decide on sterilization in response to some immediate problem, such as the occurrence of an unwanted pregnancy, without fully discussing their own and each other's feelings, may later have regrets.

4. If one or more of our children died would we want to have more?

It is generally recognized that it is impossible to replace children who have died. Each child is an individual, different from every other child. The child who has been part of a couple's early married years enjoys a place in their hearts that is different from that of the child born later in their marriage, because the intervening years have changed the parents through aging and adjustment. In this sense, producing another child is no more satisfactory than adopting a child produced by others.

5. If the husband lost his wife through death or divorce and remarried, would he wish to father more children?

Husbands often seem less concerned than their wives that they might want more children if they ever re-married. Perhaps this is because by the time a man decides he would like to be sterilized, he has reached an age when he is becoming increasingly less tolerant of small children. Also, realizing that there is a limit to how much he can earn during the rest of his life, he may understandably feel that the burden of supporting more dependents would outweigh the pleasures they might bring him.

With younger men it is not unlikely that a re-marriage would bring with it the desire to father children again. If this should occur with a man who has been sterilized, it is possible to have a rejoining operation done with a reasonable chance of success.

6.   *Are we expecting sterilization to solve marital problems?*
The changes in sexual relations which may follow sterilization are unlikely to improve marital disharmony. If there is anxiety over the possibility of pregnancy, release from this fear may enhance an already stable union. But since problems with sexual relations are often symptoms rather than causes of conflict between two persons, sterilization may or may not improve sexual intercourse, and is not likely to have any beneficial effect on other problems. The frank discussions between husband and wife which should precede sterilization, may serve as an opportunity to resolve their differences. If they have not previously taken the time to listen attentively to and consider each other's points of view, they may be surprised at the progress they can make. In some cases, however, the help of a skilled marriage counselor will be required.

7.   *If the pattern of our sexual relations changes following sterilization are we both willing to make adjustments according to our partner's needs?*
Sterilization brings freedom from fear of pregnancy and from the need to use contraceptives. At first it may seem that this cannot help but improve sexual relations. But this is not always the case. Couples who use one form of birth control for many years become accustomed to a certain frequency and pattern of intercourse. Freedom to have intercourse whenever they like may result in one or both of the partners having difficulty in adjusting. One may find the other too demanding, or may be disturbed by his or her change in aggressiveness or wish to try out different approaches. Furthermore, changing

from a method of contraception controlled by the woman, such as the Pill, or by the man, such as withdrawal or the use of condoms, to a condition in which the control has been removed from both of them, though only the man is sterile, may be upsetting to their relationship.

Preparing for and arriving at a decision to have sterilization performed can be one of the most co-operative ventures of a marriage. The decision to stop having children, and the actions taken to fulfill this decision are perhaps even more important, and require higher levels of co-operation than are needed to produce a child. Too often families just "seem to happen" without any apparent planning, and not uncommonly in spite of attempts to regulate their size. Before planning sterilization a couple should fully discuss all aspects, including their motives, their future needs, and their concerns, if any, about what effects the operation might have on their feelings about themselves and each other.

The foregoing questions and comments are intended to help people come to a decision with full awareness of what they are doing. But they should not be concerned if they cannot give definite answers to all of them. No one can be completely confident when approaching an unfamiliar situation, nor can he be certain what his feelings will be under changed circumstances. In coming to a decision a couple will recognize that there is some risk involved, simply because they are unable to predict the future. That is just a part of living. If they have done their best to arrive at a decision that seems right for themselves and their children they are unlikely to have any serious regrets no matter what the future may bring.

After a decision has been reached to have the operation, an application may be made to a surgeon to perform it. There should be a waiting period of at least two weeks before it is actually done. This gives time for reconsideration to the occasional person who, being unable to come to terms with his doubts, and fearful of being thought afraid, attempts to deny his doubts by hurrying to get the operation completed before they again immobilize him. This only compounds the problem, because after the operation he still has to deal with his old doubts, in addition to his new condition which he was not previously prepared to accept.

THOSE WHO DO NOT WANT CHILDREN

There are various reasons for not wanting to produce any children, some of which are easily accepted, and others which may seem radical. There are instances of later marriage, or of the strong possibility of producing children with congenital defects. There are those who simply cannot see any place for children in their lives and recognize they would not make good parents. For them, sterilization is probably wise and desirable. Others, who might make good parents, feel they can contribute more to society if they are free of the responsibility of raising children.

If such people are young, being sterilized may seem a very radical step to take. But if the decision has been reached after long and serious examination of all the considerations, and with the help of adequate counseling, there is little doubt that it will be a sound one. Besides satisfying their desires, a couple will be avoiding the possibility of producing an unwanted child, with all the undesirable consequences, and will be helping to alleviate over-population, with all its related problems which exist in the world today.

Since there is always the possibility they might change their minds and regret sterilization having been done, the surgeon, before undertaking to perform the operation, needs to be convinced that the partners' beliefs are strongly held. At the same time he has to accept the possibility of them having future regrets, realizing that this is far better than the risk of producing an unwanted child. Adults can find ways of compensating for their regrets, but an unwanted child has no choice. He develops in response to his environment and has no way of understanding his situation until after his personality has been molded.

Occasionally a request for sterilization comes from a young unmarried man. He might be emotionally confused and seeking to reject all responsibility, or he migh be a highly intelligent person who has worked out a plan for his life which he might well be able to follow successfully. No matter what he appears to be, he is entitled to an attentive and sympathetic hearing. A surgeon, understandably, will agree to such a request only in an exceptional case. He would probably require a long waiting period, repeated discussions and perhaps the results of a psychological examination indicating that adverse emotional reactions are unlikely to follow.

2   VASECTOMY COUNSELING

by Robert B. Benjamin, M.D.

"We want far better reasons for having children than not knowing how to prevent them."

Dora Russell

"The problem of population is the problem of our age."

Julian Huxley

In counseling couples who are considering vasectomy as a means of contraception, I have tried to play the role of resource person rather than judge. I believe the surgeon should refrain from making value judgments or decisions such as "you are *too young* to have a vasectomy" or "you *do not have enough children.*" Rather, I have described the operative procedure, its risks, and results. In addition, all patients are given two explanatory pamphlets on vasectomy. The patient and his wife then have been allowed to make a decision as to whether they believe a vasectomy would be beneficial to their marriage.

It is of considerable benefit, in order to counter the many adverse and faulty statements made about this procedure, to make some very positive statements about the vasectomy operation based on many excellent studies. It is important to inform the couple that the testes continue to manufacture sperm following this operation. It is valuable to point out that the operation does not affect the "manliness" of the man undergoing the procedure. Studies on men who have undergone vasectomy demonstrate somewhat greater testosterone production by the testes following the operation. The surgeon should always explain that orgasm and ejaculation are not impaired, and the volume of ejaculate is the same following vasectomy. One might also refer to the excellent studies which indicate that following

vasectomy, husbands and wives, on the average, have intercourse more frequently than other couples and enjoy their sex
life more. One should be completely honest about the reversibility of the procedure, now possible in over 80% of patients
desiring it. However, it is important to point out to the patient
that in *any particular individual* it may not be reversible and the
patient should be willing to accept the operation as an *irrevocable
loss of his fertility.* The surgeon should require both husband
and wife to sign consent forms at the conclusion of the consultation if they desire a vasectomy. The operation is then scheduled for a later date.

It is important to inquire into the nature of a marriage.
A brief but candid discussion of a couple's sex life is particularly important. In my experience, only a small percentage of
couples who request vasectomy will be found to have a poor
sexual adjustment. It is worthwhile to refer these patients for
marital counseling. In such marriages one may still proceed
with a vasectomy, as this has not been found, in the author's
experience, to lessen the excellent results obtained from marital counseling.

THE COUPLE WITH NO CHILDREN

In a society which demands conformity it is almost easier
to have a dozen children than to have none. Nevertheless, there
are a surprising number of married (and unmarried!) couples
who never desire children. When they are young this can be
quite disconcerting to the surgeon. They should be apprised of
all risks, and especially of all alternatives to vasectomy. Usually
one finds that they have thought the question through quite well
before coming to the consultation room. If they still desire
sterilization after being informed of all other methods of contraception at their disposal I always proceed with the operation.
The following case is illustrative:

Case No. 1. Mr. R., a Ph.D. candidate, 25 years old. Wife
is 24. Attractive, intelligent couple — referred to me by a social
agency. Married over two years. They have decided never to
have children and they dislike all three of the contraceptive
measures they have used thus far. Mrs. R. has a satisfying career

in computer programming. They are quite certain they will never desire children but, if they do, they would prefer adoption.

STERILIZATION OF SINGLE MEN

All single men requesting vasectomy thus far have been allowed to have the operation. Among the first 500 vasectomy patients there were thirteen single males. Ten years ago my convictions, or rather lack of them, were such that I referred single males to other surgeons. Experience with these earlier cases demonstrated to me that single males could utilize this procedure to help them find more meaning and happiness in life and at the same time protect society by the prevention of unwanted pregnancies. Each request is different. One patient may have frequent relationships with many women while another has a significant relationship with only one woman. Age is quite variable in this group. Because of the situational variability it is important that the surgeon point out the possibilities that may cause the patient to later regret his vasectomy. On the other hand, there are cases where it seems almost justified to perform the sterilization primarily for the protection of society:

Case No. 2. Mr. J., 23 years old, an intelligent, handsome manager of an insurance company, was referred by a private social agency. He had never been married. He heard Dr. H. Curtis Wood on the "Joe Pyne Show" and then read Dr. Wood's book *Sex Without Babies.* He had impregnated four women and arranged abortions for two of them. He loves children and is a "Big Brother" in the Big Brother Organization. However, he does not think he would ever want children of his own.

It would appear, in view of the present sexual revolution, that there will be an increasing number of single men requesting sterilization. To date all of the single men who have undergone vasectomy have been satisfied. There have been no requests for reversal.

3   HESITATIONS AND WORRIES OF 330 COUPLES CHOOSING VASECTOMY FOR BIRTH CONTROL

by Judson T. Landis and Thomas Poffenberger

The data in the present study provide some background information on 2,007 males who requested and underwent vasectomy operations in a California city and more detailed information on a sample of 330 of these men. The operations were all performed by the same surgeon, who required only that both husband and wife sign a release stating that they agreed in consenting to the vasectomy.

Most of the operations were performed between 1956 and mid-1961. All were done in a clinic located in the workingman's zone of a large central California city. The surgeon's fee was $50. The doctor suggested to patients that a sperm count be taken about one month following the operation, and this service was included in the fee. According to the surgeon, the operation involved about twelve minutes of the patient's time from waiting room to waiting room. No cases of serious complications following the operation were reported, and the surgeon had encountered no court action or threat of such action.[1] During the period covered by this study ten men requested reversal of the operation. The surgeon reported that seven of the ten reversals were successful, in that viable sperm were found in later sperm counts.

Data for the 2,007 men were taken from the card file kept by the surgeon. Limited background data had been recorded by a receptionist at the time of each operation and this was made available to the investigator. These data were placed on a code sheet and punched on IBM cards. Information made available

Paper read before the session "New Work in Fertility and Fertility Control," Annual Meeting, American Sociological Association, Los Angeles, California, August 29, 1963.

[1]Although some doctors hesitate to do vasectomies because they fear legal action, no state specifically forbids therapeutic sterilization. See Richard C. Donnelly and William L. F. Ferber, "The Legal and Medical Aspects of Vasectomy," *The Journal of Urology*, 81 (2 Feb. 1959), pp. 259-263.

to the researchers included age, date of operation, occupation, any medical reasons for having the operation, and number of children at the time of the operation. A detailed questionnaire was sent to 750 of the 2,007 patients with a covering letter from the doctor explaining the nature of the study and asking for co-operation in the study. A return envelope addressed to the doctor was enclosed. Of the total mailing, 330 usable questionnaires were returned; approximately 190 were undelivered for lack of a correct address.

Comparisons between the sample of 330 and the total of 2,007 indicate that these 330 are a representative sample of the total group. The mean age of the men in the sample was 31.0; that of the total group was 31.8. In the total group 56 per cent of the men were 31 years or younger; and in the sample group 59 per cent were this age. Ten per cent in both groups were over forty years old. In the total group 66 per cent had three or fewer children; in the sample 75 per cent had three or fewer children. Ten per cent in both groups had more than four children. The three groups of skilled, semi-skilled and unskilled workers account for 72 per cent of the total group and 71 per cent of the sample group. And finally 15 per cent of the total group and 14 per cent of the sample group gave a medical reason for the vasectomy.

Since on the basis of the material available for comparison of the total group and the sample, it appears that the sample reflects the general demographic characteristics of the total group, our detailed analysis will be of the 330 who responded to the questionnaire.

REASONS FOR HAVING THE VASECTOMY

The immediate intent of the vasectomies was, of course, to prevent future conception of children. A variety of prior experience with contraception was reported. Of the group, 53 per cent reported that the wife had not become pregnant while using a contraceptive and 39 per cent reported that she had; 8 per cent more were not certain whether or not conceptions had occurred while a contraceptive was being used. In 19 per cent of the cases the wife had become pregnant two or more times while using a contraceptive. In analyzing the responses by a number of variables (occupation, education, age, religion, marital status, and length of time since the operation), no great differences between those who had been able to control conception by means of contraceptives and plan their children and those who had not were found. The largest percentage of unplanned pregnancies occurred among those who were either under 26 years old or over 37 years old; the middle age group exhibited a lower percentage than either of these. The diaphragm, either alone or with jelly or cream, was the method most often reported by all groups as having failed, with one exception. Catholics reported greatest failure while practicing the rhythm method.

The respondents were specifically questioned on their reasons for having had a vasectomy. Only 14 per cent said that it had been for medical reasons; the most common response (64 percent) was that they had as many children as they could afford. Twenty-one percent felt that contraceptives interfered with sexual pleasure; 18 per cent, that they did not trust contraceptives; 15 per cent, that they were beyond the age where they wanted more children and 12 per cent, that their wives were reluctant to have sex relations unless they had the operation.

Professional men, men age 32 and over, and men who had been divorced were all more likely to give advancing age as their reason for wanting the vasectomy than were the complementary groups (nonprofessional, etc.). Men 31 and under and especially men 25 and under were more likely to report as their reason for the vasectomy that they could not afford more children. Higher percentages of men who had attended college stated that they did not trust contraceptives than of those with less education. Protestants more than Catholics gave a medical reason for the vasectomy while Catholics more often stated that the wife had been reluctant to have intercourse before the sterilization operation. In the group of men 38 and over the wife's reluctance to have intercourse was given more emphasis than in younger age groups. This suggests a greater fear of pregnancy at later ages. No other significant differences in the responses concerning reasons for the vasectomy were found.

Respondents were asked whether husband and wife together had made the decision to have the operation and whether they had considered a salpingectomy. Ninety-three per cent reported that they had made the decision together and 42 per cent that they had not considered the wife's having the sterilization operation. Of the 58 per cent who considered salpingectomy the predominant reasons given for finally choosing the vasectomy were the following: that it is easier for a man (78 per cent); that it is cheaper for a man (46 per cent); that they did not want to place more burden on the wife (21 per cent). Further analysis of the responses concerning reasons for the vasectomy revealed only slight differences on variables. Semi- and unskilled men and Catholics more often mentioned expense. Protestants and men over 25 more often mentioned that the male sterilization operation was easier for the male than the sterilization operation for the female.

Findings on how much deliberation the couple had put into the vasectomy decision were striking. Seventeen per cent reported that they had considered having the vasectomy for less than a month, 29 per cent from 1-6 months and 23 per cent from 7-11 months. Seventeen per cent had considered it for 1-2 years, 13 per cent for 2 or more years, and 5 per cent had considered it for five years or more. It is somewhat surprising that so little time would be given by almost half the group to deliberating before making the decision to have the operation. Analysis of the respondents on this matter revealed no consistent trends in background variables.

Inquiry was made as to fear felt over the operation. Forty-one per cent of the men reported that they had no fear at all of the operation and 53 per cent reported some fear; 6 per cent reported much fear. Fear of the operation was more likely to be reported by those men under 26 years old, those who had had the operation within the past two years, Protestants, and those who had never been divorced. Men with some college education seemed to have as much fear of the operation as did those with less than a high school education, and pro-

fessional men expressed almost as much fear as did the semi-
and unskilled workers.

The respondents were asked whether they believed a
vasectomy would lead to more freedom in having extramarital
sex relations. Nine per cent reported that they would be
more likely to be promiscuous and 11 per cent that they would
be less likely to. The largest group (57 per cent) felt that it
would make no difference and 23 per cent did not know whether
it would. An analysis of background variables revealed no
significant findings.

Detailed information was sought from the husbands
responding on why each partner in the marriage hesitated or
was worried about having the vasectomy. The men were asked
to check any of a series of 18 items indicating their own worry
or hesitation before the vasectomy. Since some of these items
were very similar we have combined them into ten items for
presentation in Table 1. The husbands were also asked to check
any of 18 items which might have caused their wives to hesitate

TABLE 1.   Percentage Distribution of 308
Vasectomized Males by Age at Vasectomy
and Reasons Why Half Hesitated or
Worried About Operation*

Causes for hesitation or worry	25 & under N=58	26-31 N=118	32-37 N=75	38 & over N=50	Total N=301**
Concern about sex drive	24.1	22.7	25.3	28.0	24.6
No more children	31.0	23.5	21.3	8.0	21.9
Concern about masculinity	3.4	5.9	9.3	18.0	8.3
Concern regarding others' opinions	3.4	1.7	4.0	2.0	2.7
Religious reasons	8.6	11.8	10.7	10.0	10.6
Thought illegal	5.2	5.9	8.0	2.0	5.6
Might run around	1.7	4.2	—	2.0	2.3
Fear of pain of operation	43.1	33.6	33.3	22.0	33.6
Couldn't start new family	36.2	21.8	16.0	10.0	21.3
Cost or finding a doctor	3.4	2.5	5.3	—	3.0
No hesitations or worries	24.1	29.4	32.0	44.0	31.6

  * Multiple-punch category: columns do not equal 100%
 ** No answer: 7

about the husband's having the vasectomy. These items have been combined in Table 2.

Table 1 breaks down the responses of the men concerning their worry or hesitation, by the ages at which they had the operation. It will be observed that approximately 32 per cent reported that they did not worry or hesitate because of any of the specific items listed, and that younger men reported more concern than older men did. The chief concerns centered around pain or fear of the operation, fear that the sex drive might be affected, concern that they could have no more children by the present wife or that they might want some day to start a new family.

When the concerns were analyzed on the basis of the background variables few differences were found. The professional-managerial occupational group reported greater fear than did the other occupational groups. Those with less than a high school education were more concerned about the effects on their sex drive than were those with more education, while those with more education were more concerned about not being able to have more children if they should wish to and about not being able to start a new family. Catholic men were much more likely than Protestant men to give religious reasons for hesitation. Men over 37 were more concerned about what might happen to their masculinity than were younger men. Men under 26 were more concerned about possible pain of the operation, that they could never have more children or start a new family if they should want to, than were men over 37.

The fears some of the men expressed about pain and the operation seem to have been unwarranted. No one reported serious pain or complications as a result of the operation and few missed work. Sixty-six per cent reported they had the operation on a week end and returned to work on Monday and 16 per cent more had the operation during the week and went to work the next day. Twelve per cent had the operation on a weekday and missed one day of work and 6 per cent more reported they missed two to five days of work. The fact

TABLE 2.   Percentage Distribution of 308
Vasectomized Males by Age at Vasectomy
and Reasons Why Wife Hesitated or Worried
About Operation*

Reasons for wife's hesitation or worry	25 & under N=57	26-31 N=115	32-37 N=76	38 & over N=43	Total N=289**
Concern with sex ability	7.0	9.6	5.4	7.0	7.6
Might run around with other women	26.3	22.6	5.4	11.6	17.3
Damage to organs	10.5	9.6	6.8	4.7	8.3
Religious reasons	12.3	16.5	6.8	9.3	12.1
Might blame her if he resented it	21.1	21.7	27.0	14.0	21.8
Might want more children	22.8	15.7	13.5	7.0	15.2
Might want intercourse too often	8.8	3.5	6.8	11.6	6.6
Wondered if a sure thing	33.3	38.3	33.8	27.9	34.6
Deny being child's father if became pregnant	22.8	27.0	13.5	9.3	20.1
Didn't worry	24.6	17.4	35.1	44.2	27.3
Suggested operation	42.1	32.2	41.9	32.6	36.7

* Multiple-punch category: columns do not equal 100%
** No answer: 19

that 54 per cent resumed intercourse from the first to the
seventh day after the vasectomy would also indicate that for
these the operation was not serious.

The check list for what the husbands thought their wives
hesitated about is given in Table 2. It will be observed that the
most frequent answer was that it was the wife who suggested
the operation. A large percentage also indicated that the
wife did not worry about *anything* relating to the operation.
The women were more concerned about whether vasectomy
was a reliable preventative of conception than about whether
the husband would lose his sexual ability. The wives were also
concerned about whether the operation might cause the husband to be promiscuous and whether, if the masculinity of the
husband should be affected, she might be blamed. These findings suggest a female viewpoint in rather distinct contrast to the
male viewpoint on the vasectomy operation.

A number of religious differences were found in analyzing wives' concerns by the background variables. Catholic men reported more frequently than Protestant men that their wives were concerned that the husbands might be promiscuous with other women, and that they (wives) might be blamed if the husband regretted the operation. More of the Catholic wives reportedly had religious concerns, and more of them suggested the operation. A slightly larger percentage of Protestant than Catholic men reported that their wives wondered whether the operation was a dependable preventative or that their wives had had no worries. Other background differences included the following: more men under 32 than men 32 and older reported that their wives feared that the husbands might be promiscuous. A larger percentage of men over 37 at the time of the operation reported that their wives had no concerns than was true of younger men, especially men under 32 (See Table 2). A larger percentage of professional men, men who had a high school education or more, and men who had had the operation less than five years ago reported that their wives worried about whether the operation was a sure preventative of conception.

SUMMARY OF FINDINGS

1. A sample of 330 men largely from the lower socioeconomic classes who had had a vasectomy as a means of birth control was studied to determine whether there were differences between men of different socio-economic-educational backgrounds in various aspects of the decision to have a vasectomy.

2. Respondents were classified on a number of social variables. In all the groups a large percentage of previous pregnancies had been unplanned and their chief reason for wanting a vasectomy was that they had had as many children as they could afford. The mean number of children in the families was three, and only 10 per cent had four or more children.

3. The predominant reason for the man's having a vasectomy rather than the wife's having a salpingectomy was

that it was easier and cheaper for the man to have the operation.

4. Almost half the group considered the decision to have the operation for less than six months before having it and slightly over 50 per cent reported no fear of the operation.

5. More than half of the men reported that they felt that having a vasectomy would not lead to a man's being promiscuous or unfaithful to his wife.

6. The men's chief concerns before having the vasectomy were their fear of pain, fear that their sex drive might be affected, and concerns over the fact that they could have no more children in the future if they should wish to. The men repored that their wives were most concerned about whether the operation would surely prevent conception, whether the husband might be promiscuous with other women, whether the wife might be blamed if the husband's masculinity was affected or if the wife should later become pregnant.

7. Analysis of the reported reasons for fears and hesitations about having a vasectomy by the background variables of occupation, education, religion, age at time of vasectomy, marital status, and time since having had the vasectomy revealed few significant differences. Religious faith and age at time of vasectomy were found to be the most discriminating of all the variables in revealing differences.

DISCUSSION

Some general questions which this study has raised cannot be answered because we do not know to what extent the 330 men have answered the questionnaire (or for that matter the 2007 men who had had the vasectomy by this particular doctor) are representative of American men. However, we do know that this study looked more closely at the lower socio-economic levels of our society than many other studies have done. Because of this, two common assumptions have been brought into question. In discussions of vasectomy it is assumed that less informed people would resist having vasectomies because they do not distinguish between vasectomy and castration. There is no evidence in this study to indicate that the grade school graduate has any more fears about vasectomy than does the man who has had some college education. Also it is sometimes thought that couples who resort to drastic measures such as sterilization are those already overburdened with large families. This also was not true of the people in this sample. They did have more children than they had wanted but they had wanted very small families.

The findings suggest that an important factor causing very young couples to agree upon the husband's having a vasectomy may possibly be how soon and how rapidly after the marriage successive children are born to them. It could be that the young couple who have two or three unplanned pregnancies in three or four years become desperate at the apparent prospect of a large family, and so resort early to vasectomy. Possibly older couples who have even one unplanned pregnancy are impelled toward vasectomy for the same reason. Our data show that the men under 26 and over 37 reported larger percentages of unplanned pregnancies in their marriages than did those 26 to 38 years old. Also, those under 26 were more likely to report as their reason for having the vasectomy that they could not afford or that they did not want more children.

REFERENCES:

Butler, Fred C., "Sterilization in the United States," *American Journal of Mental Deficiency,* 56 (2 October 1951), pp. 360-363.

Chaset, Nathan, "Male Sterilization," *The Journal of Urology,* 87 (3 March 1962), pp. 512-517.

Donnelly, Richard C., and William L. F. Ferber, "The Legal and Medical Aspects of Vasectomy," *The Journal of Urology,* 81 (2 February 1959), pp. 259-263.

Garrison, P. L., and C. J. Gamble, "Sexual Effects of Vasectomy," *Journal of the American Medical Association,* 144 (4 September 1950), pp. 293-295.

Gosney, E. S., and Paul Popence, *Sterilization for Human Betterment,* New York: The Macmillan Company, 1931.

Guttmacher, Alan F., *Babies by Choice or by Chance,* Doubleday and Company, Inc. (New York), 1959. Also reprint of "Surgical Birth Control" in *True Story* Magazine.

Landis, Judson T., "Attitudes of Individual California Physicians and Policies of State Medical Societies on Vasectomy for Birth Control," *Journal of Marriage and the Family,* 28 (3 August 1966), pp. 277-283.

Landis, Judson T., and Thomas Poffenberger, "The Marital and Sexual Adjust-
    ment of 330 Couples Who Chose Vasectomy as a Form of Birth Control,"
    Journal of Marriage and the Family, 27 (1 February 1965), pp. 59-64.
Poffenberger, Shirley B., and Thomas Poffenberger, "Interview Report of Fifty-
    six Sterilization Cases Performed at a Rural 'Camp'." *The Journal of Family
    Welfare,* 8 (September 1962), pp. 1-7.
Poffenberger, Thomas, and Shirley B. Poffenberger, "Vasectomy as a Preferred
    Method of Birth Control," *Marriage and Family Living,* 25 (3 August
    1963), pp. 326-330.
Rieser, Charles, "Vasectomy: Medical and Legal Aspects," *Journal of Urology,*
    79 (1 January 1958), pp. 138-144.
Rodgers, David A., Frederick J. Ziegler, Patricia Rohr, and Robert J. Prentiss,
    "Sociopsychological Characteristics of Patients Obtaining Vasectomies
    from Urologists," *Marriage and Family Living,* 25 (3 August 1963), pp. 331-33
Stycos, J. Mayon, "Female Sterilization in Puerto Rico," *Eugenics Quarterly,*
    1 (2 June 1954), pp. 3-9.
Weintraub, Phillip, "Sterilization in Sweden: Its Law and Practice," *American
    Journal of Mental Deficiency,* 56 (2 October 1951), pp. 364-374.
Woodside, Moya, "Sterilization and Social Welfare," *Eugenics Review,* 40
    (4 January 1949), pp. 2-7.

4 REASONS FOR WANTING A VASECTOMY

Report by the Simon Population Trust, Cambridge, England

The 1,012 men whose reactions to vasectomy are here
described are the great majority of a self-selected sample of 1,092
whose operation was mediated through the Simon Trust's Vasectomy Project. Only 80 of these men (7 per cent) having agreed
to cooperate, failed to return completed questionnaires.

The 1,012 respondents are scattered over the United King-
dom; and the questions asked are given verbatim before each of
the tables which follow. Not all the 1,012 respondents answered
all the questions. Hence the totals of some of the tables fall
slightly short of 1,012.

These questionnaires were submitted to men a year or
more after they had undergone vasectomy. In addition to the
questions, a space was left on the back page of the questionnaire
for remarks or amplifications. Many respondents here expressed
themselves freely.

The nine reasons for wanting a vasectomy shown below were listed in the questionnaire. They include an omnibus category "Other Particular Reasons." Since most people who have had as many children as they want have several reasons for not wanting more, respondents were asked to record such multiple reasons as may have influenced them in obtaining vasectomy. One thousand and ten respondents gave 3,489 reasons, thus averaging over three reasons per respondent.

In Table 1 these reasons are tabulated in a descending order of the frequency with which they were given; and in Table 2 is shown how many reasons (from 1 to 5+) were given by the 1,010 respondents.

From Table 1 (percentage column) it will be seen how variable was the frequency with which the nine listed reasons were acknowledged as operative: the range is from nearly 80 to under 4 per cent. Also noteworthy is the sharp drop from 50 to under 20 per cent betwee the fifth listed reason (failure of contraception, line e) and the sixth (line f). The first five of the listed reasons (lines a to e) were each given by more than half the sample; the last three (lines g to i) by under seven per cent or one in fourteen respondents at most.

THE TABLE HAS OTHER NOTEWORTHY FEATURES:
1. Dislike of contraception (line a), is the most widely held reason. Contraception is adopted as the lesser of two evils — the other being a fertility deemed to be excessive for the family concerned. Contraception is disliked with varying degrees of intensity ranging from a faint distaste to an aversion which may be so strong as to affect the husband's potency and cause him to prefer surgery. There may be some overlap between the responses to question a (dislike of contraception, acknowledged by nearly four-fifths of the sample) and to question e (failure of contraception resulting in unwanted pregnancy). It is reasonable for people to feel dislike for a procedure which has failed in its main purpose. (The incidence of unwanted pregnancies is of unfading interest to demographers, who would all

TABLE 1. Reasons for Seeking Vasectomy

Reasons for seeking vasectomy given by 1,010 respondents	Total number of times each reason was given	Percentage of 1,010 respondents giving each reason
(a) Dislike of contraception	802	79.4
(b) To spare respondent's wife because the operation on the male is less serious	769	76.1
(c) Financial considerations	539	53.4
(d) Health reasons affecting respondent's wife	510	50.5
(e) Failure of contraception (unwanted pregnancy)	508	50.3
(f) Other particular reasons	205	20.3
(g) Health reasons affecting respondent	64	6.3
(h) Blood incompatibility (including rhesus incompatibility)	55	5.4
(i) Fear of transmitting unfavourable hereditary conditions	37	3.7

Total Reasons: 3,489
Total Respondents: 1,010

TABLE 2.   Number of Reasons Given by 1,010 Respondents

Respondents giving:	Number	Per Cent
One reason only	68	6.7
Two reasons	170	16.8
Three reasons	275	27.2
Four reasons	296	29.3
Five or more reasons	201	19.9
*Total	1,010	100

*Excluding two men, who gave no reasons.

like to know what would be the effect on the replacement of the population if all unplanned pregnancies were eliminated.) The discovery of an ideal contraceptive — wholly reliable, harmless, fool-proof, aesthetically unobjectionable, cheap, and without side effects — would, if it were universally adopted, largely eliminate reasons a and e and would indeed completely extinguish the demand for vasectomy.

2. Another noteworthy feature of Table 1 is the part played by the respondents' concern with the well-being of their wives. Over three-quarters (76.1 per cent: line b) wish to spare their wives an operation which is more serious for them than vasectomy is for the respondents; and over half (50.5 per cent: d) were influenced by consideration for their wives' health. The term "health" has doubtless been broadly interpreted. The wife's physical health, perhaps impaired by the effects of earlier pregnancies, and her mental health, perhaps affected by fear of further unwanted pregnancies (which occurred in over half the cases: line e) certainly are involved.

3. The two questions (lines b and d) bearing upon the well-being of the wife may have overlapped in the sense that both may have been answered in the affirmative by many respondents. By contrast, Table 1 shows how relatively few men (64, or 6.3 per cent: line g) gave their own health as a reason for seeking vasectomy. Relevant to the husband's health may have been a degree of repugnance for coitus interruptus (which feeling can be intense in some men) and a degree of anxiety about failure of contraception, each or both being of sufficient strength to affect health. Again, a minority of men are prone to anxiety, which can focus itself in numerous ways. An anxiety about an unwanted pregnancy, which may not be the first of its kind, has more logic than many widespread but baseless anxieties and phobias. But however this issue may be, Table 1 shows a conspicuous drop in the incidence of the last three reasons (lines g to i) below that of the next most prevalent reason (line f) — a drop of more than two-thirds from 20.3 to 6.3 per cent.

4. Many published reports which have tabulated the reasons for which men have sought vasectomy do not take

account of how frequently multiple reasons are operative. They give but a single reason, so that the number of reasons adds up to the same figure as the number of respondents. Table 2 shows that, in our sample, only 68 (6.7 per cent) respondents gave a single reason.

Part Three ♀♂

Vasectomy: A Simple Medical Procedure for Men

1 DESCRIPTION OF AN IN-OFFICE OPERATION

by Donald J. Dodds, M.D.

To understand the method of male sterilization and its effect it is necessary to have some knowledge of male anatomy (see illustration). The male sex cells, called sperm, are like minute tadpoles with long tails. They are made in many small tubes in the testicles. These tubules come out of each testicle and join together to form one main tube, called the vas, which goes from behind its testicle up into the groin on the same side. A similar tube goes from behind the testicle to the groin on the other side. From the groins the two vasa go inside the body, behind and under the bladder, and enter the penis just after it comes out of the bladder, that is, between the legs. Each vas has a widened part, called the ampulla, close to where it ends in the penis. The ampullas are storage spaces for the sperm. The fluid which comes from the penis during intercourse is called semen. The liquid part of the semen comes mainly from a group of glands which lie around the base of the penis, called the prostate, the seminal vesicles, and Cowper's glands, as well as from the ampullas.

During each intercourse the semen which is ejaculated, or squirted out, contains a few hundred million sperm, whose combined volume is less than one tenth of the total volume of the semen. To start the growth of a baby requires only one of these remarkably small and complex organisms to enter an ovum, or egg, in the female. The ovum itself would be barely visible to the naked eye.

The sperm are dormant, and lie still until they have been ejaculated from the penis. They are moved from the testicles to the ampullas by squeezing movements of the vasa. During intercourse sperm are squeezed from the ampullas into the penis where they mix with the fluids from the semen glands, and soon afterwards they become very active. While they are in the vasa and ampullas the sperm can live for several weeks, but after they have been deposited in a woman's body, and have become active, their life is limited to from a few hours to a few days.

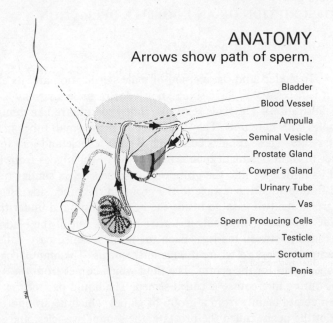

ANATOMY
Arrows show path of sperm.

Bladder
Blood Vessel
Ampulla
Seminal Vesicle
Prostate Gland
Cowper's Gland
Urinary Tube
Vas
Sperm Producing Cells
Testicle
Scrotum
Penis

The testicles have another function besides making sperm, which is to make chemicals called hormones. The male hormones are produced by specialized cells which lie between the tubules which produce the sperm. They go directly into the blood stream, which spreads them throughout the entire body. Women's reproductive glands, called ovaries, produce female hormones as well as ova. The differences between the effects of the male and female hormones account for many of the differences between men and women, including hair and fat distribution, muscle and breast development, and pitch of voice.

The sterilization operation on the male is generally known as a bilateral vasectomy. Literally this means cutting out the vas on both sides, but actually surgeons usually remove less than one and a half inches of each vas, and often do not remove any of it. The operation could be done on any part of the vas, but is generally done on the portion in the scrotum midway between the testicle and groin, since this is the part most easily reached.

THE OPERATION
Showing one method
of separating the ends of the vasa.

Location of midline incision. Often two incisions are made, one on each side.

Loop of vas tied in two places.

Vas cut, one end sewn back. Same operation done on right vas. Skin stitched.

Prior to the operation, patients who might be unduly nervous are given a sedative to help them relax. The region where the operation is to be performed, which has been shaved beforehand, is washed with a surgical cleanser. The surgeon then feels for one of the vasa. He can distinguish it from other cords by its size and firmness, since it is much harder than anything else in the scrotum. He manipulates the vas to the front of the scrotum and holds it in a suitable position under the skin. An anaesthetic solution is then injected around the vas and into the skin over the vas, using a small needle. This is the only time during the operation when the patient actually experiences pain, and it is usually no worse than an injection for tetanus, polio, or allergy. The anaesthetic takes effect in a minute or two, after which the surgeon can operate without causing any pain.

The surgery consists of making a small incision in the skin, about three quarters of an inch in length, and bringing out a loop of the vas. The loop is cut and the two ends are tied off with ab-

AFTER THE OPERATION
Sterility is not immediate because:

- Microscopic partitions in ampullas delay clearing out of sperm.
- Sperm remaining in ampullas need several weeks to become incapable of causing pregnancy.
- Rejoining can occur until scars over ends of vasa have matured.

Health and sex life is not altered because:

- Sperm, hormones and semen fluid continue to be produced.
- Sperm collect here, disintegrate and are absorbed into the body.
- Hormones continue to be secreted into the bloodstream.
- Semen fluid glands still discharge into the penis.

sorbable surgical thread. The thread takes about two weeks to dissolve, and during that time a scar begins to develop over each end, which eventually seals off the end permanently. The vas on the other side is treated in the same manner, and the skin is stitched. A support for the scrotum is worn for a few days. The operation does not interfere with urination.

In most patients there is enough freedom of movement of both vasa to permit them to be brought out through a single, mid-line incision. For the remainder a separate incision is made for each vas.

The operation lasts from fifteen to forty-five minutes depending on the surgeon and on technical differences. These come from the need to make either one or two incisions, and from various methods used to try to prevent the ends of the vasa from rejoining themselves. A piece of each vas may be removed, a layer of fascia, or sheet of tissue, may be sewn between the ends, the ends may be overlapped, one end (or both ends) may be turned and sewn back on itself, or a combination of these methods may be used. In spite of these techniques, and no matter which method is used very occasionally the ends manage to rejoin themselves.

Following the operation the effect of the local anaesthetic gradually wears off and a dull ache is felt in the region of the operation and often also in the lower abdomen. This is not severe enough to require any special medication, but a few mild pain-relieving tablets such as aspirin, or aspirin with codeine, may be used. Most men are ready to return to work, even very heavy work, two days after the operation, and those whose jobs require little standing or walking can usually return to work the day after the operation.

Sexual intercourse may be resumed after about ten days. This gives time for the skin incision to heal. If begun earlier the success of the operation is not likely to be affected, but there might be some discomfort.

by **Robert B. Benjamin, M.D.**

The patient is advised to take a bath and shave his scrotum the night before his vasectomy. He brings an athletic supporter or suspensory with him. No preoperative medication is given. After the scrotum is prepped and draped, the surgeon palpates the scrotum and locates the vas deferens on one side of the scrotum. his assistant helps him fix the vas in a relatively superficial position. Procaine is then injected into the overlying skin and into the vas and surrounding tissues. A one centimeter incision is made into the scrotal skin. After a brief dissection with a mosquito forceps the vas is grasped with an Allis forceps and brought out of the wound. Surrounding tissues are dissected away and a 3 cm. segment of vas deferens is excised between dacron sutures. In very young patients or in others for whom I feel there is a greater likelihood of regretting the procedure, a lesser amount of vas is excised, always in the straight portion, so that the chance for restoration of fertility, should it later be desired, will be about 80-90%. Bleeders are controlled with electrocautery and one or two sutures are used to close the skin. Baciguent ointment and a Band-Aid are applied to the wound. This procedure is repeated on the other side of the scrotum unless the patient has only one testis. The patient with only one testis presents a special problem which the surgeon should anticipate. My first such patient stated that since he had only one testis and vas deferens (the other having been removed because of a malignant seminoma) he expected to be charged only *half* the usual fee! I replied that since he had continued to impregnate his wife, even after having one testis excised and the entire area subjected to cobalt radiation, I had concluded that he was an unusually fertile man, would be extremely difficult to sterilize, and should our operation be successful, I had intended to charge him *twice* the standard fee. We were both happy to compromise on the usual charge.

At the conclusion of surgery the nurse supplies the patient with a reiteration of postoperative directions and also gives him a small envelope of three narcotic tablets in case he should have unusual pain. The patient then puts on his support and goes home. He is advised to rest two or three hours with an ice pack on his scrotum and refrain from any undue physical exertion for the remainder of the day. The following day he may climb trees or play football if he is so inclined. However, he is advised to refrain from sexual intercourse for six or seven days. Sutures are removed in 48 hours.

The patient continues to wear his support until he is comfortable without it — usually two or three days. Both he and his wife are advised to rely on previous methods of contraception until the first sperm count, obtained seven weeks after surgery, reveals the patient to be sterile. For additional tranquility a second sperm count is recommended five to six months after surgery. Both the patient and his wife are informed that additional sperm counts may be obtained at no additional charge at any time. This helps allay any anxiety over the possibility of an unwanted pregnancy.

RESULTS

The more important results of vasectomy cannot be tabulated. The maintenance of a happy marriage with spontaneous and happy sexual relations, the stabilization of a marriage that might otherwise have deteriorated, the magnificent change in the sex life of a couple whose previous relations were clouded by overwhelming fear of pregnancy are things that no philosopher, let alone a surgeon, can measure.

Easy to tabulate are the results of the procedure in respect to post-operative sperm counts (Figures 1 and 2). In the earlier years some sperm counts were obtained as early as two weeks following surgery. Some men were found to be fertile at this time but became sterile by the time a second sperm count was obtained. Six men were found to be fertile as a result of recanalization following the operation. All six underwent reoperation and remained sterile after the second procedure. In the first 500 patients three wives became pregnant. Two of these pregnancies occurred during the first six weeks following surgery. For this reason I now delay the first sperm count until 8 weeks after surgery and advise the use of other contraceptive measures during the interim. The third pregnancy occurred as the result of an illicit affair by the patient's wife. One of these pregnancies was terminated by an abortion obtained in Japan. I do not know the outcome of the other two pregnancies.

To date, in over 1,000 patients, no wife has become pregnant by her husband following two "negative" sperm counts. The same result has obtained in all cases where the first "negative" sperm count has been delayed until at least seven weeks following vasectomy. We now ask all couples to obtain at least *two* sperm counts. If the first sperm count is delayed until 8 weeks and is negative, I believe that no other contraceptive measures need be taken, as a vasectomy and 8-week negative sperm count provide greater "protection" than any other conventional method of contraception.

Complications have been few and minimal (Figure 3). The two patients with orchitis were treated for five days with tetracycline and obtained a good recovery in both cases. One patient developed a spermatogenic granuloma which caused him pain during intercourse. This was excised in the office under local anaesthesia with a good result. One patient who developed a hydrocele following a vasectomy had it excised.

Only one patient has desired reversal of his vasectomy. This man and his wife were Roman Catholics with five children. Unknown to me, his wife had left him and refused to live with him until he underwent vasectomy. One year following the vasectomy she stated that there must be "something sinful" about having marital relations and not having to worry about pregnancy. She then left her husband again and said she would not sleep with him until he had the vasectomy reversed! Her husband was already overburdened financially with five children and neither of them desired a larger family. This woman was severely neurotic but refused to obtain psychiatric care. Her husband was referred to another surgeon for a reversal operation. He stated that in about three months his wife would probably leave him and request that he be vasectomized again!

VASECTOMY SURVEY

RESULT OF FIRST SPERM COUNT

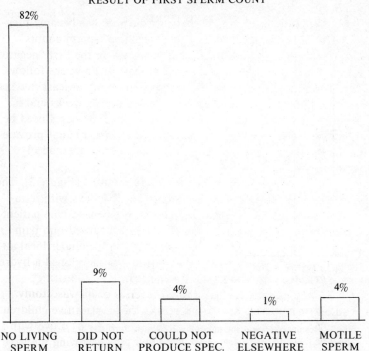

Fig. 1   Results of first sperm count on 500 patients. In earlier patients sperm counts were obtained as early as two weeks following surgery. Four percent were found to have viable sperm in the ejaculate. These fertile patients all returned for a second sperm count (see Fig. 2).

COMMENT

Thirty-five to forty percent of the children born in the United States are unwanted. Fortunately, many of these children later become "wanted." These unwanted children are an expensive social burden and frequently become involved in delinquency. The solution to this problem rests primarily with physicians. Measures other than contraception do not get to the root of the problem.

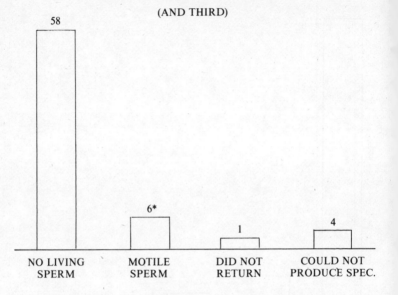

VASECTOMY SURVEY

RESULT OF SECOND SPERM COUNT

(AND THIRD)

* ALL RE-OPERATED AND THEN FOUND TO BE STERILE

Fig. 2   Results of second sperm counts in 69 men. Included are the 20 men who were found to have viable sperm on the first sperm count. Only 6 patients (1% of the total group of 500 patients) were found to have motile sperm at the second sperm count. These six patients all remained sterile after a second operation.

There is a suggestion that couples are now desiring smaller families. C. W. Truesdale, reporting in 1965 on 200 patients on whom he had performed vasectomy, noted that the average number of children in the families in his series was 4.1. In this study the average number of children per family is 3.2.

This difference may be due partly to restrictions utilized by Truesdale; he sterilized only one male who had less than two children, whereas nine percent of my patients fell into this group. The difference may also be a reflection of the difference between a rural (Glencoe, Minnesota) practice and an urban (St. Louis Park, Minnesota) practice.

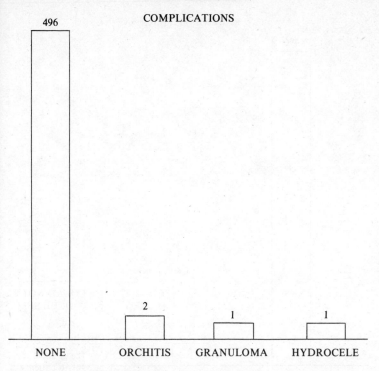

VASECTOMY SURVEY

COMPLICATIONS

Fig. 3   Complications in 500 patients following vasectomy.

Of some concern is the strong impression that the highly educated, well-to-do caucasian is more likely to request vasectomy than the less educated, poor member of a minority racial group (Figure 4). An inordinately high percentage of physicians, ministers, social workers, professors, teachers, and lawyers are found among those who have undergone vasectomy in my practice. Some method of education is needed to provide people of *all* socio-economic groups with the basic knowledge required to make an intelligent decision regarding contraception. At present only one-sixth of those who are too poor to pay for contraceptive advice and help are actually obtaining it.

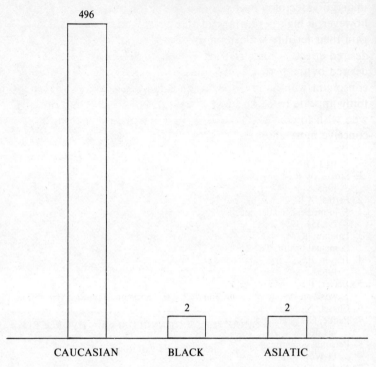

Fig. 4   Race of 500 vasectomy patients.

Religious objections are not as great as might be supposed. Analysis of the first 500 patients in this series reveals that 17% are Roman Catholic. Only 1% of the patients were Jewish. Orthodox Judaism does not sanction sterilization. However, there must be other reasons for the relatively small percentage of Jewish patients who undergo sterilization.

SUMMARY

Male sterilization following adequate counseling is a procedure having few complications. Very few males who undergo vasectomy ever desire to have the procedure reversed; however, a high percentage of those desiring reversal *can* regain their fertility with modern surgical techniques. Since the desired effect — male sterility — can be verified whenever desired by the performance of a sperm count, the procedure is consonant with happy, spontaneous marital relations. Vasectomy appears to be an ideal contraceptive measure for those who wish to continue an active sex life but do not wish to conceive more children.

REFERENCES

1. Stokes, W.R.: Long-range effects of male sterilization. Sexology, October, 1965.
2. Ferber, A.S., Tietze, C., and Lewit, S.: Men with vasectomies: A study in medical, sexual and psychosocial changes, Psychosomatic Medicine 29: 354, 1967.
3. Laidlaw, R.W., and Bass, M.S.: Voluntary sterilization as it relates to mental health. The Amer. J. Psychiatry 120: 1176, 1964.
4. Jhaver, P.S.: Surgery of the epididymis and vas. J. Indian M. A. 44: 591, 1965.
5. Jhaver, P.S., and Ohri, B.B.: The history of experimental and clinical work on vasectomy. Jour. Internat. Coll. Surgeons 33: 482, 1960.
6. Chaset, N.: Male sterilization. Jour. Urol. 87: 512, 1962.
7. Padke, G.M., and Padke, A.G.: Experiences in the re-anastomosis of the vas deferens. Jour. Urol. 97: 888, 1967.
8. Personal communication. Association for Voluntary Sterilization, Inc., 14 West 40th St., New York, N.Y. June 1969.
9. Nielsen, D.J., and Green, W.A.: Personal communication. July, 1968.
10. Mead, M.: Personal communication. Nov., 1969.
11. Guttmacher, A.: Personal communication. Nov., 1969.
12. Truesdale, C.W.: Assessment of vasectomy as means of voluntary sterilization. The Journal-Lancet (Minneapolis) 85: 155, 1965.
13. Guttmacher, A.F.: Sterilization. Nation, April 6, 1964.

Part Four ☿♂

Techniques of Female Sterilization: Breakthrough in the Out-Patient Clinic Approach

1   A CAPSULE REPORT FROM *TIME* MAGAZINE

For women there is a variety of surgical procedures. The most obvious is used on the woman who is having a baby by caesarean section, and has decided that this will be her last. Since her abdomen is already open, the obstetrician simply reaches in for the Fallopian tubes, ties them off and severs them — much as the urologist does in a vasectomy. Most surgeons also remove part of the tube. This procedure is called tubal ligation.

Equally common is the operation on a woman who has just given birth to a baby normally. Within 36 hours after the delivery, the surgeon makes a three- or four-inch incision in her lower abdomen to reach the tubes. The surgical wound is almost healed by the time the woman goes home with her baby.

In recent years, especially in Britain and Europe, gynecological surgeons have been seeking means of reaching and severing the Fallopian tubes without making a long pelvic incision. They have succeeded with the aid of the laparoscope, a tube containing a "light pipe," less than half an inch in diameter. The techniques vary in detail. At Johns Hopkins Hospital in Baltimore, Dr. Clifford R. Wheeless makes two incisions less than half an inch long just below the navel *(see diagram)*. Through one, after blowing in carbon dioxide to

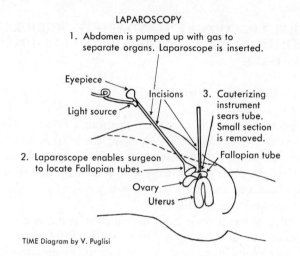

LAPAROSCOPY

1. Abdomen is pumped up with gas to separate organs. Laparoscope is inserted.

Eyepiece

Incisions

3. Cauterizing instrument sears tube. Small section is removed.

Light source

2. Laparoscope enables surgeon to locate Fallopian tubes.

Fallopian tube

Ovary

Uterus

TIME Diagram by V. Puglisi

separate the organs, he inserts the laparoscope to locate a tube. Through the second he inserts the electric cautery and a tiny surgical knife. The operation, under general anesthesia, takes about 30 minutes and allows the patient to leave the hospital the same day.

In a modified version of the operation, Dr. Alvin Siegler of New York's Downstate Medical Center makes his first incision for the laparoscope so close to the navel that no separate scar will be visible, then inserts the cautery and knife through two punctures not much bigger than those made by a heavy-gauge hypodermic needle.

The simplest development in sterilization of women, requiring only local anesthesia, is reported by Dr. Martin Clyman at Manhattan's Mount Sinai School of Medicine. He has designed special instruments that enable him to operate through an incision little more than an inch long in the vaginal

wall, reaching and tying off both tubes in about ten minutes.
This vaginal approach leaves the patient with no visible
scars, and she can go home in 24 to 48 hours after the operation.

2   TUBAL LIGATION BY STANDARD TECHNIQUES AND THE NEW LAPAROSCOPIC AND CULDOSCOPIC APPROACH

by Robert S. Neuwirth, M.D.

Female sterilization, or tubal ligation, is best done in the
post-partum period when it is technically easier to perform and
does not add much to the recovery time following birth. It
must always be done abdominally, and can be performed under
local anesthesia as the uterus is enlarged, bringing the tubes
up near the abdominal wall.

Interval sterilization on a woman who is not and has not
been recently pregnant is more complex. This is usually a
vaginal or abdominal procedure. The incision when post-
partum is usually small and near the umbilicus. The incision
when interval is made low down on the abdomen or in the
vagina behind the cervix. The advantage of the vaginal
approach is that there is no visible scar, and post-operative
hospitalization is often shorter than for the patient having an
abdominal incision. The disadvantage is that there are sometimes technical factors that make this approach difficult or
impossible.

Tubal ligation can be performed in many ways. In the
Madlener technique, probably the oldest, a loop of the tube
is lifted and a clamp placed across the loop, which is then
crushed. A surgical tie, usually catgut, closes the segment.
This technique, infrequently used now, has a relatively high
failure rate due to tubo-tubal (the tract between ends of the
cut tube) fistula formation at the site of the crush.

In the most commonly used Pomeroy technique, a loop
of tube is tied with plain catgut and the intervening segment

excised. This simple technique can be done vaginally or abdominally, and has a failure rate of approximately 1 in 200 post-partum, and about 1 in 500 for interval sterilization. The higher failure rate post-partum probably stems from the greater incidence of low grade infection in the tubes at the site of ligation. The infection predisposes to fistula formation between the separated segments of the tube.

Following failed sterilization, a pregnancy may be aborted in those states with legalized abortion, and the procedure redone if the patient desires.

Other techniques include removal of both tubes, removal of the fimbria of the tubes only, and methods of separating the cut ends of the tubes and burying them in different tissues. These methods, more complicated and time consuming, are aimed at producing foolproof tubal ligation. At the moment, the Pomeroy procedure appears to be the best balance between an effective operation and minimal complications.

Female sterilization carries more risks than male sterilization. Dr. Christopher Tietze of the Population Council reported one fatality per 3,000 operations in a collected series in 1963. The rate of death is in about the same range as the rate of death associated with pregnancy in the U.S. Most have occurred in patients with underlying medical conditions which make pregnancy, as well as sterilization, more risky. In otherwise healthy women, the operation has an extremely low mortality rate and other complications are usually minor.

After a standard abdominal or vaginal procedure, women require three to four days of hospitalization before they can manage at home alone. The rate of postoperative problems, reported at about 7 per cent, stems predominantly from wound or urinary infection. Serious complications, such as bowel obstruction, phlebitis, pulmonary embolism, and hemorrhage are rare. Ill-defined complaints, including abdominal discomfort and menstrual irregularity, are difficult to interpret since the majority of patients report satisfaction with the sterilization operation.

Operations to reverse tubal ligation are reported to be about 40 per cent successful as proved by subsequent pregnancy. However, this rate is low enough so that tubal ligation must be considered nonreversible, particularly because tuboplasties (repairs) are major and expensive procedures. Several investigators have been seeking to develop a truly reversible tubal ligation, but no satisfactory method is yet available. Nor does much information exist on the frequency of requests for reversal. The rate probably runs about one per 1,000 tubal ligations — about the same range of requests for reversal in men.

As sterilization has achieved growing acceptance, two new techniques, which attempt to make the operation easier, less costly, and potentially reversible, are rapidly gaining adherents in clinical practice. Both depend on telescopic visualization of the tubes and fiberoptic lighting. In the culdoscopic approach, the patient is placed in the knee-chest position, sedated, and given local anesthesia infiltrated into the posterior fornix of the vagina. A culdoscope, or viewing instrument, is inserted through the posterior fornix, and the tubes visualized. After removal of the culdoscope, and widening of the puncture wound, the surgeon reinserts the culdoscope, and with a special grasping instrument, brings the tubes into the vagina, where a Pomeroy tubal ligation is done. A single suture closes the wound. Patients may be discharged as early as 4 to 6 hours after the operation. Full recovery takes a few days.

The laparoscopic approach employs similar equipment but entry is made at the umbilicus. The patient, anesthetized with regional or general anesthesia, is placed on her back with legs in stirrups. The cervix is grasped with a tenaculum (toothed grasping instrument), and a cannula (hollow metal tube) locked into the cervical canal. A needle, inserted at the umbilicus, introduces carbon dioxide gas. The abdomen distends, and the laparoscope, or viewing instrument, is introduced at the umbilicus. With the tubes visualized, a special grasping, cutting, and electrocoagulating instrument is inserted in the lower quadrant of the abdomen. This instrument grasps the tube and holds it away from other structures. After electrocoagulation, the tube is transected and the procedure repeated with the other tube. Patients may be discharged as early as six hours after this operation. Full recovery takes only a few days.

Both new approaches have provided women with a much easier alternative, almost approximating the vasectomy in simplicity. Long-term experience is still limited, but they appear about as effective as standard tubal ligation.

Nonsurgical sterilization methods are also under development. In Chile, a method that repeatedly irrigates the uterus with medications eventually blocks the tubes where they enter the uterus. This is an office procedure, not requiring anesthesia, and takes only a few minutes. The side effects and complications thus far have been inconsequential. But there are two problems. First, it requires three separate monthly applications. Second, experience is small and long-range results unknown.

Female sterilization has now become an almost ambulatory procedure. Both the culdoscopic and laparoscopic techniques permit rapid recuperation to the point that the patient can care for herself within hours following the operation. Neither technique, however, is fully ambulatory. An occasional patient requires an overnight stay, more frequently with the laparoscopic approach. Both procedures require an operating room or specially designed treatment room, expensive equipment, and skilled gynecologists.

For patients in emerging countries, unfortunately, the cost of equipment and trained personnel are too high to make these operations readily applicable. Hence, we have a real need for a transcervical procedure which is safe and reliable. Such a procedure would be truly ambulatory with little or no anesthesia necessary, and it could be accomplished in a clinic or office setting offering other forms of obstetrical, gynecological, or contraceptive services. Within a few years, it is likely that it will be possible to provide female sterilization without anesthesia or an incision.

3 "TYING THE TUBES" WITH LAPAROSCOPY

by J. F. Hulka, M.D.

Over the past several years, a new permanent method of
birth control has been developed in England and America. The
new method requires no major surgery and the patient can go
home the same day as the procedure is performed. It is called
"laparoscopy," from the Greek words literally meaning "looking into the abdomen." The procedure is often done under
local anesthesia (not putting the patient to sleep) when doctors
simply want to look in the abdomen. But when the tubes are
to be sealed, the patient is usually put to sleep for about 30
minutes.

Patients asking about the procedure are first seen in the
clinic, where the decision to have no more children is reviewed
by the doctor and the couple. For this first appointment, the
doctor usually talks to both the husband and wife if the woman
is married.

This procedure is not recommended for all women who
want no more children. Sometimes previous surgery, being over-
weight, or other medical problems may mean that another
solution to her problem should be worked out. But for women
with completed families who are sure they want no more
children and do not want to use ordinary birth control methods
for the rest of their reproductive years, this method is quicker
and less expensive than the usual tubal ligation or hysterectomy. The usual tubal ligation is considered major surgery —
it requires a large incision and several days' hospitalization.
The laparoscopy method, a 15-minute procedure requiring only
one night [or less] in the hospital, is much less complicated.
Laparoscopy has been proved in thousands of British and
American women as a sensible permanent method of birth
control.

No matter which method of sterilization a couple seeks
(laparoscopy, tubal ligation, or vasectomy for the man), it
should be understood that doctors have to make the final decision whether or not they will perform the procedure. There

is *no* law which requires a couple to have a certain number of children before sterilization may be done, but any doctor who performs sterilization operations wants.to be sure that the couple requesting the procedure is mature and fully aware that this is a permanent step. Physicians feel it is their obligation to make this judgment.

After the doctor fully discusses the details of sterilization, sterilization permission papers are signed and the patient is scheduled to return for surgery. When she returns, routine laboratory work is done and she is admitted to the hospital to allow the medical and nursing staff to prepare her for the procedure, which will take place the next morning. Preparing the patient simply means that she will have a light supper and a good night's sleep. No special medication or shaving of any part of the body is required.

In the morning the patient is put to sleep in an operating room, and about two quarts of carbon dioxide (a clear gas that is safe to use with electric currents) is put into the abdomen through a special needle that is inserted just below the navel. This little opening in the skin is then made slightly larger (about as wide as a fingernail) and an instrument called a laparoscope, which is about as big around as a fountain pen, is inserted into the opening. With the use of this instrument, the surgeon can now see all the organs through the clear gas.

The tubes are between the womb and the ovaries and are smaller in size than an ordinary pencil. They are held with a special electrical instrument introduced through another, smaller opening lower in the abdomen. An electric current seals the tubes to prevent bleeding and the tubes are permanently divided. The instruments are removed, the carbon dioxide is let out, and the patient wakes up in a few minutes with two Band-Aids over her navel and her lower abdomen.

Afterwards, women may have pains in their shoulders (from the carbon dioxide gas irritations) or pain where the instruments passed through the abdominal wall. These last a few hours and are usually gone in a day. Some may have a scratchy throat from the anesthesia. Most women are ready and eager to leave the hospital two to four hours after surgery, after the anesthesia wears off. Some are too tired from the anesthesia and excitement of surgery and appreciate an extra overnight rest. There is a discharge like a menstrual flow for a day or two. By the next day, most of these minor symptoms will be gone.

Experience with thousands of these operations has taught the medical world that they are surprisingly free of long-range complications if all goes well at surgery. About one tube in 1,000 grows back together and results in a pregnancy, about the same rate as the standard tube tying operation. At the time of surgery, about one woman in 100 has an unexpected finding (abnormally located blood vessel, adhesions between the tube and other abdominal contents, etc.) which may require a standard surgical incision to complete the operation safely. Of course, this would lengthen the hospital stay if this event occurred. Other risks are always possible, but are as rare as with any other minor operation.

4 OUT-PATIENT CLINICS: THE NEW TECHNIQUES SIMPLIFY FEMALE STERILIZATION

Three Years of Out-Patient Laparascopy at the Johns Hopkins Hospital

One of the most effective proving grounds for tubal sterilization by laparoscopy on an out-patient basis is the Johns Hopkins Hospital at Baltimore, Maryland, where 1,400 procedures have been performed. The patient enters in the morning and is discharged in two or three hours. The surgery, which once took thirty minutes, now takes only ten. Dr. Clifford R. Wheeless, Assistant Professor of Obstetrics and Gynecology, reports that some cases have been done in four minutes. Part of the reason for this efficiency is the revised technique. Instead of the usual two incisions, the Hopkins surgeons now make only one incision at the umbilicus. Either local or general anesthesia can be used, at the choice of the woman. "A simple procedure," Dr. Wheeless calls it.

With all the costs of overnight hospital care eliminated, the price of laparoscopy for the clinic or ward patient is $150. The private patient pays a surgeon's fee of $150 more.

After a careful follow-up of every woman, Hopkins has found only one subsequent pregnancy in 1,400 cases. Still, Dr. Wheeless believes that the failure rate of laparoscopy must be considered about 3 per 1,000, the same rate as standard tubal ligation by the Pomeroy method. An unwanted pregnancy from failure may be terminated by abortion in states with liberalized laws.

The Johns Hopkins Hospital has enlarged its laparoscopy program through its "satellite" service in three small county hospitals outside Baltimore — a service that could serve as a model for other states in bringing out-patient sterilization to rural areas. "The fact that the procedure can be performed on an outpatient basis should make sterilization available on a broader basis, not only in university centers, but in community hospitals and rural sterilization clinics in underdeveloped countries," Dr. Wheeless states. "The method is not difficult and could be taught to paramedical personnel under the supervision of a physician in underdeveloped areas."

TWO PIONEERING PROGRAMS IN ARIZONA

Physicians in Phoenix, Arizona, have carried the out-patient approach for laparascopy one step further — a free-standing, ambulatory clinic completely detached from a hospital setting. Phoenix's "Surgicenter," founded as a private venture by Drs. John L. Ford and Wallace A. Reed, is a small unit with four operatories and a 12-bed recovery room in a quiet neighborhood of shops and churches. Its premise is to reduce the high cost of hospitalization, alleviate the bed shortage, and eliminate expensive, overnight hospitalization for patients who can be treated within a day. Along with many types of surgery from plastic procedures to eye operations, Surgicenter features laparoscopic sterilization.

The advantage of the Surgicenter concept is both financial and psychological. As Dr. Ford points out, "The idea of avoiding hospitalization, or even entering a hospital, reduces the operation markedly in the patient's mind. They feel they are on their way to recovery as they leave Surgicenter three or four hours later."

This concept should spread rapidly. "Outpatient surgery need no longer be confined to hospitals when it can be done in a well-equipped unit like Surgicenter with medical standards equal to that of a hospital," Dr. Ford concludes.

A second pioneering step has been developed by Planned Parenthood of Phoenix, combining its own extensive facilities with those of Memorial Hospital. Along with contraceptive and pregnancy detection services, Planned Parenthood has long performed 15 vasectomies a week in its clinic, located in a wing of Memorial Hospital. Recently, the demand for female sterilization rose sharply, and Dr. Harold N. Gordon, the medical director, decided to work out a cooperative plan for low cost laparoscopy with Memorial.

One morning a week, Planned Parenthood borrows an operating room from Memorial at a charge of $125 per patient. The anesthesia fee runs $50. Preoperative counselling, examination, and medication are all done at Planned Parenthood. Dr. Gordon himself performs the laparoscopy — five cases a morning, soon increased to ten. Each week Dr. Gordon invites a different obstetrician-gynecologist as attending physician in order to inculcate a widening medical circle with the principles of laparoscopy. Patients are discharged a few hours later and pay from nothing to $175, depending on their financial status.

Such cooperation between a Planned Parenthood clinic, often the focal point of sterilization applications, and a major city hospital, provides a significant model to meet the demand for low cost laparoscopy throughout the country. "Laparoscopy on an out-patient basis fills a great void in family planning," says Dr. Gordon.

Part Five ♀♂

Vasectomy: How It Affects a Man's Physical and Mental Health, Sexual Life, and Marriage

1 VASECTOMY AS A PREFERRED METHOD OF BIRTH CONTROL

Excerpts from an investigation of twenty-nine cases

by Thomas Poffenberger and Shirley B. Poffenberger

No one reported being in poor health. Five reported that their health was "better" after the operation; 24 indicated there had been no change. Twenty-two reported that the operation had had no effect upon their weight; three indicated a weight gain. No change in sleep habits or use of alcohol was reported. Twenty-seven indicated the operation had not affected their physical strength in any way; two reported it had made them stronger.

Effect upon sexual adjustment. No change in sexual desire was reported by 18, while seven indicated a "strong" increase and four indicated "some" increase since the operation.

The data indicated some increase in reported frequency of sexual intercourse after the operation, eight reporting intercourse four to five times per week before surgery and 13 indicating this frequency after the operation. Four men felt that it had made them able to sustain an erection for a longer period while the others reported no change.

Seven men indicated that as a result of the operation they were able to control the duration of intercourse more effectively, but the majority reported no change. Most of the sample, however, reported increased enjoyment of sexual intercourse after the operation. Fifteen indicated "much greater" enjoyment; three indicated "somewhat greater" enjoyment. Eleven reported "no effect." Also, 18 men reported their wives' greater enjoyment after the operation; 11 indicated "no effect."

Effect upon marital adjustment. Eight men indicated that the effect of the surgery was to make their marital life "much happier"; five reported that it had made their life "somewhat happier." Four indicated they were "much less tense" as a result of the operation.

Most of the sample indicated that they did not care if their friends knew of their operation, but six indicated they would prefer their friends did not know. Fifteen reported that they did not know how their friends felt about their operation; 14 indicated that their friends felt favorably toward it. Eighteen indicated that their friends joked about the operation, and 12 reported that it bothered them "somewhat" to be kidded.

All of the sample reported that if they had the choice to make again they would select the vasectomy as their preferred method of birth control. They also indicated that their wives would again agree to the operation.

PERSONAL INTERVIEWS
Characteristics. Detailed information was gathered from nine couples who lived in the same university community. All the husbands and most of the wives were college graduates. The men's ages were between thirty-one and fifty-three years. Five of the couples had two children; two had three, and two had four children.

Operation. Seven of the men admitted to having had fear prior to the operation. This took two forms: 1) the fear of the operation itself, and 2) its effect upon male potency. Remarks about the former included: "I wondered if it would hurt and if the doctor knew what he was doing," and "I was very uneasy about surgery on that part of my body." Remarks pertaining to fear about sustaining an erection or to having orgasm were indicated such as, "An offhand remark about the possibility of impotency scared me but I had little fear because so many people I respected had had the operation." In every case the husband had at least one close personal friend who had undergone the vasectomy and was satisfied with it. In all cases but one the husband was accompanied by one or more friends who had either had this operation previously or who would also do so at that time. The psychological support the men felt in accompanying someone who had had the operation or someone else who was going to have it was probably a significant motivating factor in determining the number of persons who finally decided to go for surgery.

The majority of the men reported no negative aftereffects from the operation, but most of them had undergone the vasectomy some time in the past, so forgetting may have been a factor. One person who had had this surgery five weeks previously gave the following report: "The first night I felt very woozy and fatigued — a dull ache that persisted for a day or two. Climbing stairs and walking was an effort. . . . My penis became black and blue as well as my testicles and this lasted two or three weeks — not badly. The first night I had discomfort although not comparable to other minor surgery. After all, it was quite mild. I had some drainage from the operation." The man who had had a vasectomy eight months before said, "I had only slight discomfort for a few days. Had surgery on Friday and went to work on Monday. It was partly psychological. Had some tenderness for about a week — actually healed very rapidly."

Two men reported more difficulty. One who had had the operation four weeks earlier said, "I've been disappointed and surprised. I have an area about the size of a dime that is still very sensitive. On one side the scar is crooked and gave me some discomfort. No pain, but it seems to me it should have healed more quickly. Eleven days after the operation I still had some discharge. That stopped and another pocket of fluid developed and this quit only four days ago. No pus but it has been tender." This man believed that some warning should be given those having the operation as to possible aftereffects. He was also concerned because the friend who went with him who had the operation at the same time reported no difficulty at all. In a follow-up interview, this formerly worried man reported that all symptoms had gone and that he felt fine.

Internal bleeding causing discoloration concerned another man, who indicated it took "a couple of weeks to go away. . . ." In summary, most of the husbands reported no difficulty, but three did express some concern about their condition following the operation.

EFFECTS

Effect of the vasectomy on the husband-wife relationship. Two questions were asked the couples regarding the effects of the operation: how it affected their sex life and what effect it had on their total marital adjustment.

Effect on sexual adjustment. Two-thirds of the sample (six husbands, six wives) said that there had been an improvement in their sex life as a result of the operation. One of the husbands and one wife said there had been no change. Two husbands had undergone the operation so recently that these couples were not able to judge any effect.

With the fear of pregnancy removed, the couples found sexual intercourse more relaxing. One husband said, "I would say that there has been a definite increase in activity. It is more soothing — removes an element of worry for my wife and me." Another husband indicated that he and his wife felt much freer: "We never realized how worry about pregnancy affected us." Still another wife said that she had not realized the effect of worry about another pregnancy until the improvement in her sexual response following her husband's operation. A husband reported, "There is a tremendous difference in the freedom we feel. My wife feels the same way."

Effect on marital adjustment. As nearly as could be determined from the interviews, all of the couples were satisfied with their marriages. As a result of this, most of them did not feel that the operation had much effect upon their total marital adjustment. Two couples felt that their marital adjustment had improved, however, and that improvement was due to a reduction in tension related to fear of pregnancy. If improvement in the sexual adjustment of the couples is considered an improvement in the total relationship, all but one wife regarded the operation positively. The latter said that the change was, "not too great but slightly negative. I still wanted another child but my husband did not want any more. I've accepted it now but it took me a while to get used to the idea that I could not have any more children. It was difficult for me emotionally and as a result there was a certain amount of resentment." This wife did feel, however, that her relationship with her husband had improved as far as their sexual adjustment was concerned. She indicated that she was "relieved not to have to use a diaphragm," and that she and her husband had sexual intercourse "more frequently and with greater pleasure" since they didn't have to worry.

Attitude toward recommendation of vasectomy. All husbands and wives with the exception of one of each said that they would recommend the operation to others. The reluctant wife said that she would advise a couple to wait, "if one is 'lukewarm.' It's such a big step. Both should be extremely for it." Most of the couples not only had no reservations but were enthusiastic when asked if they would recommend it to others.

Not all were quite as enthusiastic, however. One husband said that he would recommend it to others but hoped that these persons would not have the drainage he had experienced.

2   THE MARITAL AND SEXUAL ADJUSTMENT OF 330 COUPLES WHO CHOSE VASECTOMY AS A FORM OF BIRTH CONTROL

by Judson T. Landis and Thomas Poffenberger

A questionnaire study was made of 330 couples who had chosen vasectomy as a means of birth control. The couples gave economic considerations as important in their decision to choose sterilization and to have vasectomy rather than salpingectomy. The respondents reported great improvement in their sex life following the operation; and, in retrospect, almost all were glad that they had had the vasectomy.

This paper will explore the marital and sexual adjustments of 330 American couples in which the husband had had a vasectomy. The data for the study came from two sources. The first was the card file of a physician who had performed 2,007 vasectomies between 1956 and 1961.[1] This file contained minimum background data — including date of the operation, the age of the husband at the time of the vasectomy, his occupation, the number of living children, and the reason given for having the vasectomy. A questionnaire was mailed to a sample of 750 of the men whose records were representative of those who had had the operation over the past several years. A covering letter from the doctor accompanied each questionnaire, explaining the nature of the study and asking the former patient to cooperate. The return envelope was addressed to the doctor. Of the 750 questionnaires mailed, 330 usable ones were returned. Comparison of the 330 men who returned the completed questionnaires with the total 2,007 men was made on certain items, indicating that on these items the responding group was comparable to the total group. The sample of 330 was weighted with people from the working classes; 71 per cent were in this

Summary of paper read before the Research Section of the Annual Meeting of the National Council on Family Relations, Denver, August 1963.

[1]For a detailed report on the data on the 2,007 men, see Thomas Poffenberger, "Two Thousand Voluntary Vasectomies Performed in California: Background Factors and Comments," *Marriage and Family Living,* 25 (November 1963), pp. 469-474.

category. This fact was paralleled in the educational breakdown of the sample: six per cent were college graduates; 41 per cent, high school graduates; and 36 per cent had less than a high school education. The sample was weighted toward Protestants (72 per cent, compared to 19 per cent Catholic men and 24 per cent Catholic women) and Caucasians (97 per cent). In national origin, the sample was mostly American (72 per cent). Fourteen per cent were West European; 12 per cent, Spanish-Italian-Mexican; and two per cent, Oriental. Both men and women tended to be young; 59 per cent of the husbands and 69 per cent of the wives were less than 32 years of age. The men tended to be in the early years of marriage: 44 per cent had been married less than seven years; 88 per cent, less than 15 years. They tended to have small families (mean number of children was three), although they had more children than they had actually wanted. Seventy-eight per cent of the men had been married only once.

FINDINGS

Major reasons for having the vasectomy. In response to the question as to why they had had the vasectomy, 64 per cent said that they had as many children as they could afford, and 15 per cent reported that they were beyond the age for having more children. Eighteen per cent reported that they did not trust contraceptives, and 12 per cent said that the wife was reluctant to continue to have intercourse unless the husband had the operation. Twenty-one per cent gave as their reason that contraceptives interfered with sexual pleasure. Only 14 per cent gave a medical problem as the reason for the vasectomy.

Over 90 per cent of the couples had decided together to have the vasectomy. Chief reasons given by the men for having the vasectomy rather than the salpingectomy were that it is easier for the man (78 per cent), that it is cheaper (47 per cent), and that they did not want to place more burden on the wife (21 per cent).

Marital adjustment after the vasectomy. One-third of the husbands reported that their relationships with their wives had improved since the operation, and they attributed this largely to improvement in their sexual adjustment. More than half of those who felt that the marital relationship had improved (60 per cent) mentioned removal of the fear of pregnancy, 17 per cent reported that the wife enjoyed sex more because she was more relaxed, and 13 per cent reported that they now had no arguments over sex or the use of contraceptives.

THE SEXUAL ADJUSTMENT

Resumption of intercourse. More than half (54 per cent) of the couples resumed intercourse within the first week after the operation, 25 per cent more within the second week, and the remainder during the third week or later. Normal living was interrupted little by having the vasectomy. Sixty-six per cent of the men had the operation on a weekend and returned to work on Monday, 16 per cent had the operation on a week day and missed no work, 12 per cent missed one day of work, and six per cent missed from two to five days of work.

Change in sexual desire. To the question, "What change have you noticed in your sexual desire since the operation?" 60 per cent reported no change, ten per cent reported a strong increase, 28 per cent reported some increase, and 2 per cent reported some decrease.

In studying the variables, it was found that the greatest change reported in sexual desire was by religion. Of the Catholic men, 52 per cent reported either strong increase or some increase in sexual desire after the vasectomy, while only 35 per cent of the Protestant men reported increased desire. Another significant factor appeared to be how long ago the operation had taken place. Of those who had had the vasectomy more than five years ago, 26 per cent reported an increase in sex desire, while 41 per cent of those who had had the operation less than a year ago reported increased sex desire. It may be that those who had the operation more than five years ago were reporting the long-time effects of the operation upon sex desire, while those who were closer to the operation were reporting their immediate reactions. Possibly the latter immediately after the operation were in a state of mind to enjoy a new freedom from contraceptives. However, a more significant factor here may be age. Analysis showed that it was the men of 25 and under at the time of the vasectomy who reported the greatest increase in sexual desire.

Frequency of intercourse before and after vasectomy. Each respondent was asked, "How frequently have you usually had intercourse before and since the operation?" A very wide range in frequency was reported by the respondents. Approximately 14 per cent had coitus three times per month or less, and 16 per cent had coitus four times a week or more. For the entire group, frequency tended to be stepped up after the vasectomy. The modal group both before and after the vasectomy was the group reporting two to three times per week (approximately 50 per cent), but approximately ten per cent of those who had coitus one time per week or less moved into the two-to-three-times-per-week group, and approximately ten per cent of those in the two-to-three-times-per-week group moved into the four-or-more-coituses-per-week group. This movement upward in frequency of coitus was characteristic of Catholics, men under 26 years old, and those who had had the operation most recently. The percentage of Catholics who had coitus four or more times per week increased from 20 before to 39 after the operation, the percentage change for men under 26 years was from 25 before to 44 after, and the percentage change for those who had had the operation within the past year was from 12 before to 29 after.

Enjoyment of sexual intercourse. Each respondent was asked to rate how the operation had affected his and his wife's enjoyment of sexual intercourse. The large majority reported that there had been a great increase in enjoyment of the sexual act. Forty-six per cent of the husbands reported that their enjoyment was "much greater," and 47 per cent reported that their wife's enjoyment was "much greater"; 24 per cent more of the husbands reported enjoyment "somewhat greater" for themselves; and 31 per cent, "somewhat greater" for their wives.

No change in enjoyment was reported by 28 per cent of the husbands for themselves and for 19 per cent of their wives. Only two per cent of the husbands reported less enjoyment for themselves, and one per cent reported less enjoyment for their wives.

Have the operation if given another chance? All but one per cent would recommend the vasectomy to a friend or would choose to have the operation again if they had the choice to make again. The investigators were interested in the cases (only four) in which the men reported that they would not have a vasectomy if they had a second choice. In these cases, the responses seemed to reveal serious fears concerning loss of masculinity. The investigators do no more than conjecture whether such fears were related to the operation or were of long standing and were more openly recognized after the operation provided an explanation for feelings of inadequacy.

3   MEN WITH VASECTOMIES: A STUDY OF MEDICAL, SEXUAL, AND PSYCHOSOCIAL CHANGES

by Andrew S. Ferber, M.D., Christopher Tietze, M.D., and Sarah Lewit

Responses to questionnaire interviews of 73 men who had undergone vasectomies are discussed, and summary tables presented. The questions cover personal characteristics, the operation itself, motivational factors, and outcome of the operation. Analysis of the outcome includes pre- and postoperative physical health; sexual behavior; psychosocial adjustment factors — including marital, job, and community relationships, and concern over children; satisfaction with the operation; and social behavior with regard to the operation. On most of these questions the respondent was also asked to evaluate his wife's condition, behavior, or attitude. Medical aspects of the vasectomy and postoperative sperm tests are also discussed.

The basic assumption of the present study is that, aside from eliminating the ability to deliver sperm, vasectomy can yield consequences that constitute the psychosocial sequelae of having decided to sterilize oneself. We sought to focus on several questions:

1. How many men and their wives had better, unchanged, and worse outcomes on major sexual, psychological, and social parameters? The self-reports of respondents in prior follow-up studies[1-7] indicate largely favorable outcomes, although a few "bad" outcomes have also been reported.

2. What are the characteristics of those who have "bad" outcomes? Can we develop predictive criteria for subjects who should not have vasectomy? Several detailed post-facto clinical reports in the literature point out instances of sexual pathologic and psychopathologic conditions in men who had undergone vasectomy and attribute the precipitation of symptoms to the operation.[1, 8, 9]

3. What are the typical "trouble spots" before, during, and after the operation, and how can the physician best assist the patient in coping with them? The trouble spots were: how men decide to have a vasectomy and what doubts make them hesitate, postoperative morbidity, results of sperm tests, typical anxieties surrounding sexual questions, and the possible trauma associated with revealing the operation to others.

We analyzed the data in two ways: (1) description of the demographic characteristics, the medical course, and the sexual, psychological, and sociological outcomes; and (2) correlation between demographic and motivational characteristics (independent variables) and various outcome scores summarizing responses in the areas of physical health, psychosocial adjustment, and sexual satisfaction of husband and wife (as well as coital frequency) as dependent variables. However, no statistically significant correlations were found between the independent variables and outcome scores because of the small numbers of unfavorable outcomes involved.

METHOD AND MATERIALS

Study outline. The present study is a follow-up of 73 urban-area men who had applied to the Association for Voluntary Sterilization (AVS) for assistance in finding a physician to perform a vasectomy, and who had had the operation in the preceding five years.

The interviewers were male residents in psychiatry at medical schools located within the interview areas. A modest honorarium was paid for each completed interview, which lasted about two hours. Residents in psychiatry were preferred because it was felt that by training they could exercise greater skill and judgment in obtaining answers to questions of a highly personal and emotional nature.

Letters were sent to the men to be interviewed asking for their cooperation in a study which was "to gather information which will be useful to other men who may consider a vasectomy, to family counselors who give advice on the matter, to physicians who perform the operation, and to hospitals in the formulation of policies." The men were assured that all information would be held in the strictest confidence.

Questionnaire. The questionnaire was developed in collaboration with a number of urologists, psychiatrists, psychologists, and family counselors who were asked to submit lists of questions. The responses were pooled and a draft sent out for critical comments and suggestions. On this basis, a revised draft was tested in the New York City area by one of the authors (A.F.), and further changes made. The final questionnaire, consisting of 96 questions, was divided into six segments: personal characteristics, the operation itself, motivational factors, general health, sexual health, and psychosocial adjustment.

Although we believe that the respondents told us how they felt, it should be pointed out that all responses are expressions of the respondent's opinion, bearing a complex and unassessable relationship to his real attitudes. Test-retest reliability was not studied. The questionnaires were coded so that an answer which was only slightly positive was coded as "no change" while even a slight indication of negation was given a negative value. The evaluation of responses and the assigning of code values were the responsibility of the senior author.

Subjects. Primary self-selection and persistent attempts to obtain a vasectomy (often without the help, or even in spite of the disapproval, of their own physicians) characterized the population. This motivational factor may account for the large proportion of favorable results and, also, differentiates the population from the populations studied by Ziegler and others. [1-7, 10, 11]

The 73 men in the study had made their applications to the AVS during the five-year period from 1956 to 1960, with about three-fourths in the last two years of the period. Close to one-half of them lived in the New York City area and the rest were scattered throughout 10 urban areas in the Northeast, Middle West, and Far West. Rather less than one-half requested financial assistance from the AVS.

In addition to the 73 respondents, 12 men who had received letters refused to be interviewed, of whom 8 filled in a brief questionnaire stating that they were satisfied with the operation but did not wish to be interviewed. Four men failed to respond. This does not appear to be a high ratio of refusals considering the nature of the inquiry and the socioeconomic characteristics of the respondents.

Measured characteristics. Table 1 shows the distribution of the 73 respondents by various demographic, cultural, and socioeconomic characteristics at time of interview. More than one-half of the men were between 35 and 44, and somewhat more than one-half had been married at least 10 years. None of the respondents was childless, and the great majority had at least 3 children. Most of the men (90%) were white. Somewhat more than one-half of the men stated that they were Protestants, about 1 in 5 was a Roman Catholic, 1 in 10 Jewish, and the remainder was divided between "other faiths" and "no religion."

About one-third of the men had had at least 1 year of college, and one-half possessed high school educations. More men were in professional, managerial, and technical occupations than in any other occupational category; only 2 were in unskilled manual occupations.

A comparison of the socioeconomic characteristics of interviewed men with the same characteristics in the urban population of the United States (according to the 1960 census) reveals two major differences: (1) Men in the professional and managerial occupations were overrepresented among the interviewed group, and those in the semiskilled and unskilled occupations were underrepresented, which points to the subjects' superior economic and educational position. (2) The number of children expected in an urban population of the occupational, ethnic, and age distribution of the interviewed group, according to census data, was about two-thirds of the number observed (2.3 per couple compared with 3.9 per couple), indicating a greater fecundity, or a less successful use of birth control, or both. In general, age differences between husbands and wives tended to be somewhat greater than among urban couples in the census.

TABLE 1. Distribution of Demographic, Cultural, and Socioeconomic Characteristics

Characteristic	No. of Respondents	Characteristic	No. of Respondents
Total	73	Religion	
Age		Protestant	36
Less than 35 years	21	Roman Catholic	15
35—44 years	39	Jewish	8
45 years and older	13	Other	14
Duration of marriage		Church attendance	
Less than 5 years	9	3 times a month and more	33
5—9 years	24	Once a month to a few times a year	21
10—14 years	22	Once a year or less	8
15 years and longer	18	Never	11
No. of children		Education	
1 and 2	10	Elementary school: 8 years and less	12
3 and 4	39	High school: 9—12 years	37
5 and 6	22	College: 13 years and more	24
7 and more	2	Occupation	
Race		Professional, managerial, technical	28
White	64	Clerical and sales	9
Nonwhite	9	Skilled manual	17
		Semiskilled manual	17
		Unskilled manual	2

MOTIVATING FACTORS

Reasons stated. One of the questions asked applicants by the AVS is the reason for requesting a vasectomy. One-half (37) of our sample of 73 men stated that they had inadequate economic resources; a slightly smaller number (32) mentioned emotional factors; and a still smaller number (30) offered reasons related to health — either their own or their children's. Seventeen (an average of 4 in 17) stated that they wanted a vasectomy because of previous contraceptive failures. At the time of interview, respondents gave the following answers to the question as to why they changed from other methods of birth control to a permanent one:

Didn't trust other methods	53
Finality of decision	28
Pleasure criteria	22
Anxiety over possible failure	14
Other reasons	1

The number who indicated that they did not trust other methods of contraception (53) exceeded the number who had experienced failures of contraception (48). Of the 73 men in the sample, 71 stated that they had used birth control methods prior to the operation.

Decision influences. Thirty-eight men had learned about vasectomy through professional channels, family members, or friends, and the remaining 35 through various mass media — particularly through articles published in popular journals (see Bibliography). Twelve stated that the operation had been suggested as a "good idea" by professional persons; 11 attributed the suggestion to friends or members of the family. Three felt that they had been *urged* to have the operation.

A majority (43) of those seeking the operation did not discuss it with their physicians, or stated that they had no family doctor. Sixteen were discouraged by their family physicians and sought the operation elsewhere. Only 14 men reported that their family doctors were in favor of the operation.

All 73 men reported that they had discussed the operation with their wives. The responses were:

Agreed	69
Male dominant	9
Female dominant	3
Disagreed	4

"Agreed" means that both parties concurred in the decision; "male dominant" means that the wife complied passively; and "female dominant," that the husband complied passively with the wife's decision. Four women did not agree to the plan and their husbands proceeded unilaterally.

The respondents were asked why they, rather than their wives, had undergone the sterilizing operation. The responses were:

More physical trouble for wife	38
Physician's refusal	16
More family disruption	5
More expensive	5
Other reasons	5
Not considered	15

Forty-eight (2 in 3) respondents had not discussed their plans with friends. Of the 25 men who had, 19 reported an enthusiastic reaction; 3, a neutral reaction; and 3 stated that their friends were opposed.

Twenty-nine men (2 in 5) stated that it took less than 2 weeks for them to decide to have a vasectomy; a somewhat smaller number (24) took more than 2 months; and the remaining 20 men decided in more than 2 weeks but in less than 2 months. Sixteen men had doubts about the operation, which delayed their decision, and 22 were worried or afraid before the operation. Fifty-seven stated that they had had no doubts and 51, that they had not been worried or afraid. The doubts expressed were: (1) the same sort of feeling one would have before any operation; (2) concern about the effects of the operation on their psychosexual status (e.g., "I would feel less of a man," "it might injure my manhood," "it would make me impotent or curb any sexual desire"); (3) projection of fear onto the wife (e.g., "my wife might leave me because I could

no longer have kids"); (4) realistic anxieties about a childless
future — especially in connection with the possibility of remarriage; and (5) religious scruples.

Further light was thrown on the decision making process
by answers to the question: "Do you feel that you have made
a personal sacrifice in having a vasectomy?" Six stated that
they had made a personal sacrifice. Some saw it as a sacrifice
of a capacity to have children, stressing only the loss to themselves. Others emphasized the sacrifice for someone else
— the wife or the whole family.

RESULTS
Medical aspects. Fifty-nine of the 73 operations were
performed in a physician's office, and 14 in a hospital, among
which 6 patients required 1 day of hospitalization, and 8,
2 or more days. A majority of the men (40) did not spend any
days at home after the operation; 9 stayed home for 1 day;
and 24 for 2 or more days. Local anesthesia was used in 65
cases, and general anesthesia in 8.

No pain during the operation was experienced by 52 men,
while 21 reported pain. Severe complications following the
operation were reported in 3 cases: 2 ambulatory wound in-
fections and 1 bilateral scrotal hematoma that became infected and required drainage, with the patient hospitalized.
In addition, 15 men reported minor complications (e.g., swelling
of the testicles), most of which lasted for 2 weeks or less.
The men were asked to give their subjective estimate of the
discomfort experienced during the operation, compared with
anticipated discomfort. Thirty-four reported the operation was
"as anticipated," 21 found it less unpleasant, and 18, more
unpleasant than expected.

Success in preventing pregnancy. In 70 of the 73 cases,
no postoperative pregnancy occurred, while in 3 cases, pregnancy had occurred. These 3 failures illustrate the need on the
part of the physician to make the patient aware that postoperative sperm tests must be made.

In one case of reported failure, the wife became pregnant 14 months after the operation. The man had not had any sperm tests because he "thought the operation was successful" and he "was probably too lazy." He also failed to return for treatment of a wound infection in the immediate postoperative period, again because of "laziness." In another failure, pregnancy occurred 3 months after the operation. The man had had his last sperm test 1 month after the vasectomy. A subsequent vasectomy proved successful. The third case of failure involves a man who continued to have positive sperm counts after two vasectomies. This man is now using condoms and is, understandably enough, disillusioned about the vasectomy procedure.

Postoperative sperm tests. In spite of the importance of postoperative sperm tests, 13 men reported that they did not have any, and 19 reported their last test had been made less than 1 month after the operation. In 18 additional cases, sperm tests were made 1-2 months after the operation, and in 22 cases, 2 months and more after the operation. Only 1 sperm test had been made in 33 cases, and 2 or more, in 26. For one man, no information on sperm tests was available.

The reasons given by the 13 men for not having sperm tests were: not being told about them, laziness, and embarrassment at having to masturbate (which can easily be avoided by the use of condom specimens obtained during coitus).

Resumption of sexual activity. The time interval between the operation and the resumption of sexual activity was as follows:

4 weeks and more	30
2-4 weeks	25
1-2 weeks	13
3-7 days	4
Less than 3 days	1

Fifteen men reported transient discomfort on one or more occasions during intercourse; all but two ceased within three months. The two men reported a tenderness in the testicles for 6-12 months during vigorous intercourse.

OUTCOME PARAMETERS

The outcome questions on the questionnaire almost all took the form of asking each respondent to compare his own or his wife's condition, behavior, or attitude at the time of the interview with the same variables retrospectively. Thus, each respondent served as his own control and set his own base line.

The areas chosen for investigation for possible change were: (1) physical health; (2) sexual behavior; (3) psychosocial adjustment factors — including marital, job, and community relationships, and concern about children; (4) satisfaction with the operation; and (5) social behavior with regard to the operation.

Physical health. Most of the respondents (68) stated that their health was excellent or good, and only 5 judged their health as being "fair" (Table 2). "Fair" health was assigned to a somewhat larger proportion of wives (14); one husband reported his wife in poor health. Compared with their health prior to the operation, 11 men reported changes for themselves, and 23 men for their wives. Of the 11 men who reported changes in health, 6 felt that the changes were for the better and 5 for the worse. The respondents felt that their wives' health had improved in 22 cases and had worsened in 1 case.

TABLE 2. Husband's Report of Own and Wife's Pre- and Postoperative Health Status

	Husband	*Wife*
	Health at Time of Interview	
Excellent	40	20
Good	28	38
Fair	5	14
Poor	—	1
	Compared with Preoperative Health	
Better	6	22
Same	62	50
Worse	5	1

Few of the men felt that any changes in their own health were attributable to the operation. Two of the 6 in better health and 1 of the 5 in worse health attributed the changes to the operation. On the other hand, 13 of the 22 men who reported an improvement in the health of their wives felt that the change was related to the operation. Many of the improvements referred to mental health, e.g., "my wife doesn't worry herself crazy before her periods any more," and "she no longer has anemia and fatigue from all the babies in so few years."

The psychiatrist-interviewers' estimates of the general level of psychopathology referred more to character and to chronic aspects than to acute anxiety or depression at the time of the interview. These estimates can be summed up as follows:

Severe psychopathology 4
Moderate psychopathology 32
Well-integrated 37

This distribution approximates estimates of mental health found in samples of the general population.[12] Four men had a history of prior psychiatric treatment; one had treatment after the operation and one had treatment both before and after it. However, no systematic correlation could be demonstrated between psychiatric status at the time of interview and outcome on sexual and other parameters.

A summary of postvasectomy changes in "physical" habits such as smoking, appetite, etc., included in the study appears in Table 3. Weight changes (5 lbs. or more) were reported as follows: more, 13; same, 56; less, 4; no change, 0.

TABLE 3. Habit Changes after Vasectomy

Use or Degree

Parameter	More	Same	Less	No Change
Sleep	4	69	0	0
Smoking	5	42	4	22
Alcohol	2	49	4	18
Appetite	3	67	3	0
Exercise	10	49	4	10

The data on health seem to indicate an average population which changed little and randomly after vasectomy. The improvement in the health of the wives is worthy of comment. It runs a gamut from decreased premenstrual anxiety, through the psychosomatic borderlands of less fatigue and lethargy, to improvement in varicose veins, all of which seem clearly attributable to not being pregnant frequently. No support was found for the notion that a wife may fall sick as a conversion phenomenon after the sterilization of her husband. Of the 5 men who reported a setback in their health, 1 developed Hodgkin's disease within a year of his vasectomy and was preoccupied with the possibility of some connection between the two. The others saw no connections between the operation and any deterioration in health. The validity of these data is limited by the fact that single interviews cannot reveal unconscious conflicts.

TABLE 4. Husband's Report on Changes in Own Sexual Satisfaction

Factor	Much More	Little More	No Change	Little Less
Feeling of freedom and decreased inhibition	10	40	22	1
Satisfaction with coitus	6	49	15	3
Duration of ejaculation and strength of orgasm	4	10	45	14*
Control over ejaculation	1	17	46	9
Ease and strength of erection	2	6	58	7†

*Includes 1 man who reported much shorter and weaker ejaculation and orgasm.
†Includes 1 man who reported much more difficult and weaker erections.

Sexual behavior. Because of the frequent concern of patients and physicians with the effect of vasectomy on sexual behavior, this area was scrutinized and analyzed with particular care. Data are reported for individual items, and two scales were constructed for male and female satisfaction and were correlated with independent variables.

Although the men were on the average four years older at the time of the interview than they had been at the time of the vasectomy, the mean coital frequency increased from 8.4 to 9.8 times per month, and the median changed from 10.3 to 12.6 times per month. On the basis of data reported by Kinsey and his associates, a decline of 1.2 in mean monthly coital frequency might have been expected in this age interval.[13]

Somewhat more than two-thirds of the men (50) stated that they felt freer and less inhibited sexually than before the operation, and somewhat less than one-third (22) reported no change (Table 4). One stated that he felt less free. According to the men's self-rating of "over-all satisfaction with coitus" after the operation, three-fourths (55) were more satisfied, and one-fifth (15) reported no change. Three men stated that they were less satisfied.

The self-ratings on duration of ejaculation and quality of orgasm, and on control over ejaculation were similar, with about three-fifths of the men reporting no change, between one-fifth and one-fourth reporting improvement, and the remainder (between one-fifth and one-tenth) reporting deterioration. With regard to the men's self-evaluation of the quality and ease of erection, four-fifths of the men stated that no change had occurred, while almost equal numbers of the remainder (8 and 7, respectively) reported either an improvement or a worsening in the quality and ease of erection.

Since the interviews were conducted with the husbands, only the husbands' evaluation of their wives' sexual satisfaction, which may or may not differ from their wives' own evaluation, can be presented here. Three different criteria were used as measures of sexual satisfaction.

1. Close to four-fifths of the husbands (57) reported that their wives felt less inhibited and freer sexually, one-fifth (15) were unchanged, and one wife was reported as being more inhibited (Table 5).

2. Thirty-six men reported that their wives reached climax more easily, 35 reported no change, and 2 men reported a lessened ability to reach climax on the part of their wives.

3. Close to two-fifths of the wives (29) were reported by their husbands as initiating love play leading to coitus more often than before the operation, somewhat less than three-fifths (42) as not having changed, and two as initiating love play less often.

According to their husbands, most women who improved on any one item improved on either or both of the other two items, and none of them decreased her satisfaction on any other item. A distribution of individual responses shows that only nine women were reported by their husbands as experiencing no change on all three items. Three women were reported by their husbands as having decreased their satisfaction on one or more items and none of the three showed improvement on any item. Three men and three women were less satisfied with their sex lives after the operation, according to the respondents' statements.

The men were asked questions on other types of sexual behavior, such as nocturnal emissions, daydreams, masturbation, extramarital coitus, homosexual activities, and whether they experienced fantasies about their genitalia being mutilated or cut off. Because of the infrequency and the variable nature of both the phenomena and their perceptibility, the responses did not lend themselves to quantitative analysis. They are discussed here because questions on these subjects are often raised in considering the outcome of vasectomy operations.

We were especially interested in the question on extramarital coitus because of the widely circulated rumor that men who are sterilized become promiscuous. Only one man reported increased extramarital coitus. He had been having an affair before the vasectomy and was less fearful about it afterward. Responses to this question from other men were: "Just after the operation I thought I would be a big Don Juan, but that passed away soon and I'm faithful to my wife." "I think less about other women than I did, I guess it's because I'm more satisfied now." "I have fewer fantasies about other women." "I used to have frequent fantasies and some affairs before the vasectomy, but none since. Probably because my wife seems to have changed."

TABLE 5. Husband's Report on Changes in Wife's Sexual Satisfaction

Factor	Much More	Little More	No Change	Little Less
Feeling of freedom and decreased inhibition	13	44	15	1
Ability to reach climax	8	28	35	2
Initiation of love play	5	24	42	2

One man reported an increase in masturbation, inexplicable to himself. Ideas, dreams, or thoughts that connote or mention genital mutilation were reported by several men. As outlined below under *social behavior,* it is our belief that such ideas must occur in all men undergoing the procedure.

Psychosocial. More men noted improvements in their wives' tension levels than in their own. Two-thirds of the wives (49) were reported by their husbands as being less tense compared with only two-fifths of the husbands (31). More than one-half of the men (40) reported no change in their own tension levels, while one-fourth (19) reported no change for their wives. Greater tension was reported for 2 husbands and for 5 wives.

Forty-six men (about 2 in 3) reported that they considered their relations with their wives prior to the operation better than most. Ten men felt that, prior to the operation, they did not get along with their wives as well as might be desired. All but two of the men questioned felt that this relationship had either remained the same or improved.

Most men reported no postoperative change in their ability to get along with their fellow workers (67), in their work enjoyment (65), and in their feelings of job security (63). Improvement in all three of these sectors was reported by 6, 6, and 7 men, respectively. Two men reported decreased enjoyment of their work, and three men, a lessening of their feeling of job security.

Fifty-three reported an increase in their feelings of overall happiness, emphasizing such factors as peace, stability, decision making, and the possibility of planning for the future.

Two men reported themselves as less happy. The remaining 18 men experienced no change in their self-assessment of their own happiness.

Sixty-five of the respondents stated that the operation had not increased their concern over their children, while 8 reported that it had.

POSTOPERATION ATTITUDES

Satisfaction. In spite of the variety of responses on various factors, 72 of the 73 men stated that, given the chance, they would have the operation again. The only man who said that he would not do so had already undergone two unsuccessful operations. Of the 73 men, 71 stated that they would recommend the operation to others. The two negative responses came from men who feared to make a recommendation because then "they would know I have had one."

Social behavior. In spite of the statement of most respondents that they would recommend the operation, only 35 had actually done so. An examination of the responses to the question regarding whether the respondent cared whether other people knew that he had undergone a vasectomy revealed that one-half (36) did and one-half (37) did not. Forty-eight men had told members of their family and their friends that they had been operated on, and 25 had not told anyone. Among the reasons given for not wanting others to know were: "what they would say; they are Catholics" (15); "because it's none of their business" (19); and shame (4).

The inquiry was an especially charged one. Some interviewers observed that many subjects flinched and showed tension when asked — even those who said they didn't care. It seemed clear that most men assumed a loss of status attendant upon sterilization, and while willing to deal with their own internal self-critique, were reluctant to face the disapproval of others. Some of the reported reactions of persons told about the vasectomy were: "People think it's a form of castration and affects potency." "My brother-in-law thought it unmanly. My Catholic friends said, 'How could you?' " "My brother said, 'If I had

one, I'd turn into a fairy. In a few years, I wouldn't have any
organs left.' " "My friends are generally interested and think it's
a good idea."

Some of the reasons advanced by the respondents for not
telling others about their vasectomy were: "Some men will fear
change in sex life." "People have prejudices. Would influence
their opinion of my masculinity in some way." "People will
make fun of you." "I'm a Catholic. They'd think I was bad."
"In-laws would blame my wife for forcing me into it." "My wife
thinks others would want affairs with me if they knew."

These responses seem to highlight several points. We
feel vasectomy does stimulate infantile fears and fantasies of
castration, impotence, and concomitant decline in self-esteem.
Many responses about telling people seem to be externalizations
onto a vague "other" of a man's negative feelings about himself
having had the operation. Most of these men, we feel, successfully cope with these fantasies stimulated by the operation and
do not develop overt psychosexual pathology. However, some
men fail to cope with their fantasies, and present cases where
psychosexual difficulties are traced to and blamed on vasectomy.
From a different angle, the social stigma attached to this operation is still quite high. It stimulates fantasies in others, such as
the ones respondents report hearing from people they have told
about the matter.

It appears to us that many difficulties could be avoided
by widely circulating, in popular and medical literature, the
known results of vasectomy to allay the fears of both physicians
and the general public; by stressing strict confidentiality in all
professional dealings with men seeking or undergoing vasectomy;
and by warning the men of the possibility of others having
critical attitudes towards them, suggesting that they be circum-
spect in talking about the operation. Such advice from a physician can help the men cope with the required psychological
adjustments.

DISCUSSION
The findings of general improvement on sexual and psychosocial parameters after vasectomy parallel those of several

other postoperative interviews and questionnaire surveys.[1-7]
The especially positive results our respondents report may have
to do with the high motivation of our sample in seeking this
operation.

What is the relationship of sexual and psychosocial
pathology to an antecedent vasectomy, and how high are the
chances that difficulties will occur? Two published reports that
emphasize this relationship are those of Erickson[8] and Johnson.[9]
Erickson's six cases are gathered from his psychotherapeutic
practice. He describes men who chose the operation for clearly
symbolic and self-mutilative reasons. Johnson's sample of men
was drawn from those already admitted to a VA psychiatric
hospital.

We agree with some of the conclusions of these authors:
that vasectomy is perceived by all men, on some level, in some
way, as a castration. We believe this attitude is supported by
our data on reactions of friends and relatives told about the operation, reasons given by respondents for not telling, worries
before the operation, and the heightened defensiveness shown
by respondents when being questioned about the meaning of
the operation.

We differ on the following crucial point: the relative psy-
chopathogenicity of the operation as such. We consider master-
ing the psychodynamic factors of "I will be sterile, castrated,
no good," as one of the tasks a man must go through during adjustment to a vasectomy. The changed self-image is only one of
several interacting psychological and social motives, including
the sense of mastery and relief at having taken one's destiny
into one's hands; the achieved control of a fertility that was becoming more a curse than a blessing; the loss of fear of further
pregnancies, etc. Our data indicate that the overwhelming majority of our respondents have been able to cope with the general
task adequately, and report an overall higher level of satisfaction
with life. Johnson's and Erickson's cases came from groups already psychologically decompensated.

Who demonstrated "bad" or equivocal outcomes, and
what can a study of their cases tell us about indications for denying a request for voluntary sterilization? Three men stated

that they felt less satisfied with their sexual lives after the operation. Each had a pre-existing potency difficulty that was aggravated after the operation. One reported his wife much more satisfied with their mutual sex life after the operation; the second felt there had been no change and the third had the only wife who was reported by her husband as much "worse," in her sexual expression.

Our clinical impressions were that the strongest contraindication for vasectomy is disagreement with one's wife over its advisability. Only four of our men had disagreed with their wives. Two of these showed our two worst results in terms of sexual behavior. A third was a man who, while stating his sexual life was the same, gave evidence of increased chronic neurotic tension and worry, and whose wife still held his lack of trust in her against him. The fourth subject in this group was a man whose sex life was more bound up with his mistress than with his wife. We infer that sterilization as an attempt to salvage a failing marriage seems to carry a bad prognosis.

Still another contraindication mentioned in literature is an admitted assent to the operation on the basis of another's urging. However, of the three cases of this type in our study, only one subject was rated as a bad male sexual outcome and the other two reported increased sexual satisfaction and increased happiness. It is therefore proposed that the effects of "being urged" be further investigated.

Along the same line, the possibility of a poor outcome among men seeing the operation as a personal sacrifice was also investigated. Of the six men who reported such feelings, all six reported increased sexual satisfaction, and five of the six, better psychosocial adjustments.

Of the five men with a history of prior psychiatric treatment, none had equivocal or "bad" outcomes on any parameter. Four men who showed sufficient psychopathology at interview to be diagnosed as showing severe psychopathology reported increased sexual satisfaction for themselves and their wives and improved psychosocial adjustment. We also conclude that religion, education, number of children, history of psychiatric treatment, and psychotic symptoms per se do *not* carry a poor psychosocial prognosis.

SUMMARY

A total of 73 men who had applied for a vasectomy to the AVS and who were interviewed 1 to 5 years after the operation, reported as follows:

1. Seventy anatomically successful operations and 3 failures.

2. No change in their own physical health, and a slight tendency toward improvement in the health of their wives.

3. A significant increase in coital frequency at an age when the frequency for the general population is declining.

4. Fifty-five (3 of 4) men more satisfied with intercourse, 15 no change, and 3 less satisfied.

5. Sixty-one wives reported by husbands as more satisfied with sexual intercourse, 9 no change, and 3 less satisfied.

6. Improvement on psychosocial parameters of self and wife's tension levels, relations with wife, and overall happiness were reported by between one-fourth and one-half of the husbands. Most of the rest, unchanged; some deterioration on each of these parameters reported by from 2 to 5 men. Work relationships remained unaffected.

7. Seventy-two men would make the same decision again; the one dissenter had had two operative failures.

8. Disagreement with wife over the desirability of sterilization seemed to favor development of later psychosocial pathology.

9. Evidence is presented that these men and their friends and relatives hold stereotyped attitudes equating vasectomy with being castrated and made inferior, and that the good results indicate adequate coping with these psychological factors by a large majority of the respondents.

REFERENCES

1. Dandekar, K. After-effects of vasectomy. *Artha Vijnana* (Gokhale Institute of Politics and Economics, Poona, India) 5:212, 1963.

2. Garrison, P. L., and Gamble, C. J. Sexual effects of vasectomy. *JAMA* 144:293, 1950.

3. Landis, J. T., and Poffenberger, T. The marital and sexual adjustment of 330 couples who chose vasectomy as a form of birth control. *J Marriage and the Family* 27:57, 1965.

4. Phadke, G. M. Vasectomy. *J Indian Med Ass* 37:241, 1961.

5. Poffenberger, S. B., and Sheth, D. L. Reactions of urban employees to vasectomy operations. *J Family Welfare* 10:7, 1963.

6. Poffenberger, T., and Poffenberger, S. B. Vasectomy as a preferred method of birth control: A preliminary invesigation. *Marriage and Family Living* 25:326, 1963.

7. Ziegler, F. J., Rodgers, D. A., and Kriegsman, S. A. Effect of vasectomy on psychological functioning. Paper presented at the Annual Meeting of the American Psychosomatic Society, Philadelphia, May 1965.

8. Erickson, M. H. "The Psychological Significance of Vasectomy." In *Therapeutic Abortion.* H. Rosen, Ed. Julian Press, New York, 1954.

9. Johnson, M. H. Social and psychological effects of vasectomy. *Amer J Psychiat* 121:482, 1964.

10. Rodgers, D. A., Ziegler, F. J., Rohr, P., and Prentiss, R. J. Sociopsychological characteristics of patients obtaining vasectomies from urologists. *Marriage and Family Living* 25:331, 1963.

11. Rodgers, D. A., Ziegler, F. J., Altrocchi, J., and Levy, N. A longitudinal study of the psycho-social effects of vasectomy. *J Marriage and the Family* 27:59, 1965.

12. Srole, L., Langner, T. S., Michael, S. T., Opler, M., and Rennie, T. A. C. *Mental Health in the Metropolis: the Midtown Manhattan Study.* McGraw-Hill, New York, 1962, p. 216.

13. Kinsey, A. C., Pomeroy, W. B., and Martin, C. E. *Sexual Behavior in the Human Male.* Saunders, Philadelphia, 1948, Table 56, p. 252.

BIBLIOGRAPHY

Stokes, W. R., Long-range effects of male sterilization, *Sexology,* October 1965.

Goodman, W., Abortion and sterilization, *Redbook,* October 1965.

Surgery-voluntary sterilization, *Time,* January 15, 1965.

Ridgeway, J., Birth control by surgery, *New Republic,* November 14, 1964.

Brenton, M., The most controversial method of birth control, *Coronet,* July 1964.

Anonymous, The operation that stops pregnancy, *Real Romances,* June 1964.

Guttmacher, A. F., Facts and arguments — sterilization, *The Nation,* April 6, 1964.

Laidlaw, R. W., Birth control, *New York Herald Tribune,* February 15, 1964.

Rague, J. R., Voluntary sterilization, *Med World News,* December 20, 1963.

The male operation, *Newsweek,* September 16, 1963.

Guttmacher, A. F., I just can't face having another baby, *True Story,* November 1959.

4 VASECTOMY: FOLLOW-UP OF A THOUSAND CASES

The Simon Population Trust

QUESTION 1. *Did you have any particular fear or anxiety beforehand?*

TABLE 1. Fear Beforehand in Relation to Type of Anesthetic

Fear or Anxiety   *Type of Anesthetic*

	General		Local		Total	
	Number	Per Cent	Number	Per Cent	Number	Per Cent
(a)	(b)	(c)	(d)	(e)	(f)	(g)
None	279	47.1	181	43.5	460	45.6
Average*	302	50.9	228	54.8	530	52.5
More than Average	12	2.0	7	1.7	19	1.9
Total	593	100.0	416	100.0	1,009	100.0

*As before a minor operation or dental extraction.
The total of 1,009 excludes two men who did not answer the question and one man who declared that he had had no anesthetic.

It will be seen that the respondents' recorded reactions to the two types of anesthetic differ less than might have been expected. No fear or anxiety was felt by 47 per cent of respondents in anticipation of a general anesthetic and none was felt by 43.5 per cent before a local anesthetic. Fears were what might have been expected, "average" in slightly more than half of both groups, and "more than average" in a small minority of about 2 per cent (19 respondents among over 1,000). There is little to choose between the two types of anesthetic in the matter of the preliminary fears and anxieties they evoke.

QUESTION 2.   *After-effects. Was the operation itself followed by immediate disagreeable after-effects?*

TABLE 2. After-effects.

Immediate Disagreeable after-effects	Type of Anesthetic					
	General		Local		Total	
	Number	Per Cent	Number	Per Cent	Number	Per Cent
(a)	(b)	(c)	(d)	(e)	(f)	(g)
YES	180	30.4	146	35.1	326	32.3
NO	412	69.6	270	64.9	682	67.7
*Total	592	100.0	416	100.0	1,008	100.0

*Excludes three men whose answers were incomplete and one man who declared that he had had no anesthetic.

It will be seen that over two-thirds of the respondents (67.7 per cent, column g) reported that they had had no disagreeable after-effects. Such effects as were experienced by the remaining third (326 men among 1,008: column f), though mostly, medically speaking, trivial, calling for little or no time off, were slightly more numerous among recipients of a local anesthetic (35.1 per cent: column e) than among those of a general anesthetic (30.4 per cent: column c). But as in the matter of anticipatory fears and anxieties, the difference in the incidence of unfavorable after-effects between the two types of anesthetic is too small to establish a definite superiority of one type over the other in this respect.

Of the above-mentioned 326 men who reported disagreeable after-effects, thirty-three merited serious attention. The back-page notes show that 13 of the 33 reported postoperative local infection and 12 others reported haematomata. One man mentioned a scrotal swelling six weeks, and another a testicular swelling six months, after the operation. Four men experienced epididymitis. There was a solitary case of a subsequent coronary thrombosis thought by the patient's doctor to be merely coincidental. These 33 men who mentioned after-effects which called for attention constitute a small minority of 3.1 per cent, which should be compared with the majority of over two-thirds (67 per cent) who suffered no after-effects.

Nine men required a second, and one a third, operation before they were regarded as satisfactorily vasectomized.

QUESTION 3. *Days off work?*
"For how many days were you off work after the operation?"

In tabulating the answers to this question the opportunity was taken of relating the type of anesthetic to the working time lost.

TABLE 3. Days off Work Related to Type of Anesthetic

Days off Work	*Type of Anesthetic*					
	General		*Local*		*Total*	
	Number	Per Cent	Number	Per Cent	Number	Per Cent
(a)	(b)	(c)	(d)	(e)	(f)	(g)
None	182	31.0	229	55.7	411	41.2
One	109	18.6	62	15.1	171	17.1
Two	106	18.1	43	10.5	149	14.9
Three	61	10.4	24	5.8	85	8.5
Four-Five	56	9.5	21	5.1	77	7.7
Six-Eight.	30	5.1	16	3.9	46	4.6
Nine plus	43	7.3	16	3.9	59	5.9
Total	587	100.0	411	100.0	998*	100.0

*The total of 998 men excludes eleven men who did not give the number of days off work, two men who did not give the type of anesthetic and one who declared that he had had no anesthetic.

The figures which appear in this table are of interest. They show that, in this sample, substantially more time was lost by men who were operated under a general than under a local anesthetic. Of those who had had a general anesthetic, three in ten (31 per cent: column c) had lost no time off work compared with over half (55.7 per cent: column e) of locally anesthetized men.

These differences are not entirely easy to interpret. Several factors are doubtless involved. In our view they do not signify that, for vasectomy, a general anesthetic is more incapacitating than a local. The differences in time off work are more likely to reflect the varying attitudes of surgeons. Some believe that, after most operations, patients do best if they get back to work as quickly as possible; others, more cautious, favor generous periods of convalescence. It may be that a spirit of surgical caution inclines many surgeons to prefer, for vasectomies, a general to a local anesthetic. The patient, moreover, may take more seriously an operation performed under a general than a local anesthetic and may take more time off for the former. (It was shown in the preceding table that, in our sample, immediate disagreeable after-effects occurred slightly more frequently in locally anesthetized men (35.1 per cent) than in generally anesthetized men (30.4 per cent). Some surgeons hold that, after the operation, a day and a night in bed reduce the risk of hematoma.)

By design the name of the surgeon was omitted from the questionnaire. But we know how many surgeons were concerned in the 1,012 vasectomies of our sample; and we know how many of these surgeons usually do one type of operation as against those who are prepared to vary the type of operation to suit the patient's preference and means. We are inclined to think that the surgeons here concerned mostly confine themselves to a single type of operation, particularly those who favor the general anesthetic.

We conclude our comments on the last four tables, and on Table 4 below, with a general observation. In respect of anticipatory fears, of disagreeable after-effects, of periods off work, and of willingness to recommend the operation to others, there emerges from our comparison of the two types of anesthetic no definite conclusion as to which is generally preferable.

We think it probable that surgeons will get the best results with the anesthetic they prefer. This conclusion, we believe, holds for the numerous vasectomies, running into millions, performed by many surgeons in camps and elsewhere in Asian countries.

QUESTION 4.   *Effects on Health, Sexual Life, and Marriage?*
"What Have Been the Effects of the Operation on the Following?"

(1) Yourself	(2) Your Wife	(3) Both
General Health No change Improved Deteriorated	Exactly the same questions	Harmony of Marriage No change More harmonious Less harmonious
Sexual Life No change Improved Deteriorated		

Of the above three questions, the responses to the first two are tabulated in Table 4, those to the last in Table 5.

TABLE 4. Effects on General Health and Sexual Life

Effects on Health and Sexual Life	*General Health*				*Sexual Life*			
	Respondent		*Respondent's Wife*		*Respondent*		*Respondent's Wife*	
	No.	%	No.	%	No.	%	No.	%
	(a)	(b)	(c)	(d)	(e)	(f)	(g)	(h)
No change	895	88.4	694	68.8	255	25.4	202	20.0
Improved	115	11.4	313	31.0	740	73.1	801	79.4
Deteriorated	2	0.2	2	0.2	15	1.5	5	0.5
Total	1,012	100.0	1,009*	100.0	1,010*	100.0	1,008*	100.0

*Excluded from column c, total, one divorced man and two men who did not answer question.
Excluded from column e, total, one man who did not answer question.
Excluded from column g, total, one divorced man and three men who did not answer question.

The above table is probably the one which would most interest the medical or lay reader who has an open mind on the merits of vasectomy.

In respect of the effects of the operation on *general health,* it will be seen that while a minute fraction only of husbands and wives reported a deterioration (two husbands and two wives among over a thousand couples), more wives (31 per cent: column d) than husbands (11.4 per cent: column b) reported improvements. This improvement of nearly a third of the wives can scarcely be attributed to physical causes; relief from anxieties must have been chiefly responsible. One of two men (Table 4: column a) who reported deterioration mentioned a disturbance of bladder function and the other complained of "regular backaches" after the operation, but admitted that his sex life had improved. It is impossible to say whether these complaints are *propter* or merely *post* vasectomy. The two women (column c) who complained of deterioration in general health gave no details.

The effects of the operation on sexual life are more conspicuous than those on general health. The figures are striking. Among men 73 per cent (column f), and among women over 79 per cent (column h), report improvement in their sexual lives — nearly three in four men and eight in ten women. By contrast fifteen men (1.5 per cent: column e) and five women (0.5 per cent: column g) reported deterioration. The back-page comments here throw a litle light. Of the fifteen men, one was undergoing radiotherapy for some presumably grave condition and two were under psychiatric care at the time of the operation. Another, while recording that his sexual life had deteriorated, declared that "marital harmony was unimpaired." Four men declared that, despite sexual deterioration, they had no regrets and would recommend the operation to others. One reported an "emotional" but not a physical decline. Two others attributed the deterioration to extraneous stress factors. One man had been referred by a psychiatrist in the vain hope that his own vasectomy would cure his wife's frigidity.

Of the five wives who reported a deterioration in their sexual lives, four put the trouble down to loss of libido in their husbands and the fifth attributed her own loss of libido to the onset of the menopause. Thus it will be seen that, as in the assessment of the effect on physical health, the operation of vasectomy can, in its bearings on sexual life, be wrongly blamed for unfavorable after-effects.

But the numbers of these unfavorable effects are small and the assessments are subjective in the sense that they are made by the respondents themselves. It will be interesting to see how these results compare with those of later follow-up inquiries.

The position can be summarized as follows: In respect of the effects of the operation on physical health there was no change in nearly 90 per cent of men and nearly 70 per cent of women. Among the remainder, improvements were over 50 times more numerous than deteriorations among men and over 150 times among women. In respect of the sexual life, there was no change among a quarter of the men and a fifth of the women, while among the remainder just under 50 times more men and over 150 times more women reported improvements than reported deteriorations.

QUESTION 5.   *Effects on Harmony of Marriage?*

TABLE 5. Harmony of Marriage

Harmony of Marriage	Number	Per Cent
No change	426	42.2
More harmonious	579	57.3
Less harmonious	5	0.5
Total	1,010*	100.0

*Excludes one divorced man and one who did not answer the question.

These simple figures call for little comment. A change for the better (579 couples) occurs over 100 times more frequently than a change for the worse (5 couples). Reports of a change for the better (57.3 per cent) were appreciably more numerous than reports of no change (42.2 per cent). Hence in this sample a majority of the marriages gained in harmony through the husband's vasectomy. Of the five respondents reporting a decline in marital harmony only one gave particulars — a loss of libido in the husband.

QUESTION 6.   *Recommendations to Others?*
"Would you recommend vaso-ligation to others placed like yourself?"
Again this question has been used to test the general acceptability of general versus local anesthesia.

TABLE 6. Recommendation to Others

Would respondent recommend operation to others?	Nature of Anesthetic					
	General		Local		Total	
	Number	Per Cent	Number	Per Cent	Number	Per Cent
Yes	585	99.0	409	98.8	994	99.0
No	6	1.0	5	1.2	11	1.0
Total	591	100.0	414	100.0	1,005*	100.0

*Excludes one divorced man, two who did not give the nature of the anesthetic, and four who did not answer question about recommendation.

Again the figures call for little comment. Over 98 per cent of the sample would recommend vasectomy to others. In this attitude recipients of general and local anesthesia do not differ. None of the eleven who would not recommend the operation to others expressed regrets insofar as they themselves were concerned. One reason was shyness. Another was that they did not feel that they had sufficient authority to discuss the matter with others.

QUESTION 7.   *Regrets?*
"Do either of you have regrets about the operation?"

TABLE 7. Regrets

Regrets	Respondent		Respondent's Wife	
	Number	Per Cent	Number	Per Cent
Yes	6	0.6	14	1.4
No	1,004	99.4	989	98.6
Total	1,010*	100.0	1,003*	100.0

*Total of Respondents excludes two men who did not answer the question. Total of Respondents' wives excludes one divorced man and the wives of eight men who did not answer.

Regrets are recorded by six men and by fourteen wives. In two cases both husband and wife expressed regrets. In one of these marriages a child had been lost shortly after the operation. The other couple had been warned by their doctor that there would be "psychological repercussions" and this proved to be correct.

Of the husbands expressing regret one stated that his sexual life had deteriorated. Another, while expressing regret, stated that his sexual life had improved. Another (already mentioned as suffering from a disturbance of bladder function) stated that "on the credit side, there is at least freedom from worry and a certain return to spontaneity in sexual relations."

Of women expressing regret, one had had a miscarriage after her husband's operation. Two gave no reason for regret but stated that their sex life had improved. Three others expressed "slight" regret but reported greater marital harmony. Two gave their reasons for regret as "emotional" and one stated that her husband's sterility had reduced her libido. One woman declared that she would have children continuously "if it were feasible." Thus some 99 per cent of respondents had no regrets.

QUESTION 8. *Later Follow-up*
"May we write to you again in about 18 months?"
Of 1,012 respondents, 998 (98 per cent) said yes. Permission was refused by 24 respondents, mostly on the grounds that they were emigrating or could not give a future address.

SUMMARY
This report gives a follow-up of 1,012 men who were vasectomized through the mediation of the Simon Population Trust in 1966 and 1967. Questionnaires had been sent in 1967 to 1,092 vasectomized men who had consented to fill them in.

Of these 1,092 men, 80 (7 per cent) failed to act, so that the report is based on the responses of 1,012 men — a 93 per cent sample.

The report consists of two parts which respectively deal (Part A) with the sample and its social features, and (Part B) with the operation of vasectomy: why sought; type of anesthetic; physical after-effects; effects on general health, sexual life, harmony of marriage, and later regrets.

The predominant reason for seeking vasectomy was dislike of contraception. Fifty-nine per cent of the operations were performed under general anesthesia, 41 per cent under local. Such changes as were brought about by the operation on general health, sexual life and marital harmony were conspicuously favorable: in over half the cases there was no change. But where changes were reported, they were for the better about fifty times more frequently than for the worse.

Ninety-nine per cent of the respondents would recommend the operation to others.

5   SPERM TESTS AFTER VASECTOMY

by Joseph E. Davis, M.D., and Matthew Freund, Ph.D.

Following vasectomy, either the man or woman must continue to use contraception for a period of several weeks to several months until the physician is certain that the patient's semen has been rendered aspermic (free from motile sperm cells). The persistence of sperm cells for as long as a year has been reported in a few cases. For safety, therefore, most urologists require the patient to return to his office for one, and possibly two, semen tests in the months after vasectomy.

Since the patient may undergo some anxiety about an unwanted pregnancy in this period, we have run further studies in our laboratory to increase the efficiency of determining aspermia. Using a technique of determining consecutive semen specimens following vasectomy, we have found that the end point for the disappearance of sperm can be pinpointed in a rapid and consistent manner. The patient collects his specimens immediately after the operation. The rate of disappearance of sperm from the ejaculate follows a constant percentage of decrease. Each ejaculate contains about one third the number of sperm in the previous ejaculate. With this quick and reliable technique, we believe the patient can be relieved of doubts about his sterility in a matter of weeks rather than months.

Our data on aspermia after vasectomy, however, in no way contradict the possibility that the sperm ducts, severed by the operation, may recanalize or join together again a few years later. To detect this possibility, however rare, most urologists advocate reexamination of the semen at about a year and two years following vasectomy.

For further information, see Matthew Freund and Joseph E. Davis, "Male Sterilization — Effects on the Male Reproductive System," *Medical Gynaecology and Sociology,* Vol. 5, No. 4, 1970, pp. 7-9; Matthew Freund and Joseph E. Davis, "Disappearance Rate of Spermatozoa from the Ejaculate Following Vasectomy," *Fertility and Sterility,* Vol. 20, No. 1, January-February 1969, pp. 163-170; and Joseph E. Davis, "The Consequences of Vasectomy," *Medical Counterpoint,* Vol. 3, No. 3, March 1971, pp. 50-51.

Part Six ♀♂

Female Sterilization: How It Affects a Woman's Physical and Mental Health, Sexual Life, and Marriage

1 FOLLOW-UP OF 186 STERILIZED WOMEN
by Barbara Thompson and Dugald Baird, M.D.

Follow-up of 186 women two to nine years after sterilization showed that eight regretted being sterilized. In contrast, 15 women regretted not being sterilized earlier. Forty-nine women had been sterilized in conjunction with termination of pregnancy, and two of them regretted only the termination. Most women who had post-partum sterilization were satisfied (90%); these were usually debilitated women with four or more children. The results were least satisfactory when the grounds for sterilization were specific medical, psychiatric, or obstetric conditions alone, since a quarter of these women would have liked more children. Since sterilization, coitus had been less satisfactory for 21 women, and 44 reported gynecological complaints. The problems of interpretation are discussed. Every aspect of a woman's health, marriage, and family life needs to be considered before sterilization is performed since individual circumstances, attitudes, and motivations are so very diverse. The vast majority of women, including some who reported disadvantages, were enthusiastic advocates of sterilization. For some couples, sterilization is likely to remain the most satisfactory solution for family limitation.

Sterilization is being performed with increasing frequency in women in Britain, yet the long-term effects have seldom been investigated. Since sterilization is a procedure for family limitation, attitudes to it are bound up with attitudes to family size, contraception, and therapeutic abortion, which depend on religious and moral beliefs; cultural behavior, education, and aspirations. But how do women react to sterilization? How many women regret being sterilized? Does it lead to promiscuity? These and many other questions need to be answered in assessing whether the advantages of sterilization outweigh the disadvantages.

Some follow-up studies have been done, and Ekblad (1961) in reporting his psychiatric investigation on Stockholm women, gives a summary of major series from Europe, U.S.A., Japan, and Puerto Rico. Problems of population selection and definition, different approach, and emphasis make direct comparisons impossible. But although the conclusions often differ in detail, all workers reported that while the majority of sterilized women were satisfied, a few did regret the operation.

POPULATION AND METHODS

An increasingly liberal policy on sterilization developed in Aberdeen in the 1950s and this has been maintained. Follow-up has not been systematic, but in 1955-66, five groups of these women, 186 in all, were interviewed. All had been married and living with their husbands at the time of sterilization, which was done between 1948 and 1960. Table 1 gives details.

Three of the interviewers were medical social workers who visited the women in their homes. This includes one of us (B. T.) who followed up women in groups A, B, and C. Group E *(a)* women were interviewed by a cytologist when they attended for cytological screening. All the interviewers wished to find out what the women thought about the advantages or disadvantages of sterilization and if they had any regrets.

Each woman had been a patient at the Aberdeen Maternity Hospital at some time, and 80 per cent of the women had been sterilized there. The same medical staff had sterilized the remaining women in the gynecological ward of the Aberdeen Royal Infirmary.

TABLE 1.   Description of Five Groups of Sterilized Women in the Follow-up Study

Group*	Description	Date of Sterilization	Interviewed after Sterilization		Pre-operative Home visit
			Years Later	No. of Women	No. of Women
A	All women sterilized in Aberdeen Maternity Hospital in 1 year	1948	9	14	2
B	All women sterilized primarily for reasons of D. & M. in Aberdeen Maternity Hospital in 1 year	1951	4	16	8
C	Women who had cooperated in research projects	1950-60	2-10	11	11
D	Women who had been visited at home when sterilization was being considered	1956-58	8-10	61	61
E	Women who had accepted an invitation to attend for cervical smear test	1958-60	2-4	—	—
	(a) Interviewed at clinic			65	0
	(b) Visited at home			19	19
	Total			186	101

*Excluded from the original series in groups A, B, C, and D are 20 women. 11 had left Aberdeen, 3 could not be traced, 3 had died of causes unconnected with sterilization, and information was incomplete on 3 women. Group E represents 70% of the original series but no information is available on the remainder.

Routine hospital records provided a considerable amount of social and medical data, especially since many of the women had attended during earlier pregnancies. Details were much more extensive, particularly on the marital relationship, family aspirations, and domestic circumstances, for 101 women who had been visited preoperatively either because an obstetrician had asked medical social workers for detailed reports on selected women who requested sterilization or, between 1956 and 1958, when medical social workers had visited as many as possible of the remaining women who were being considered for sterilization.

Type of operation. Sterilization was performed by tubal ligation except in 3 women with gynecological lesions on whom hysterectomy was performed. Forty-nine women were sterilized in conjunction with termination of pregnancy. These included the 3 women who had a hysterectomy. Termination was performed by hysterectomy in 45 women and by dilatation and curettage in 1. Tubal ligation was carried out on 24 women after delivery by caesarean section; 102 women were sterilized within a few days of vaginal delivery, and the remaining 11 women were readmitted specifically for tubal ligation.

Reasons for sterilization. When a virtually irreversible measure of family limitation such as sterilization is being considered, all aspects of a woman's health, marriage, and family life must be taken into account. In some cases specific medical considerations are of primary importance — e.g., when a woman is having a second or third caesarean section or when she has a severe medical or surgical condition. Less clearly defined illness associated with poor or difficult social circumstances makes the decision on sterilization more controversial and more dependent on the doctor's attitudes. The written consent of both husband and wife is also required before sterilization is performed.

The indications for sterilization are often multiple but they can be divided into broad groups.

Medical — Serious disease, normally of heart, chest, or kidneys, which makes childbearing dangerous to life or health.

Psychiatric — Severe mental disturbance necessitating psychiatric treatment, which makes further childbearing inadvisable.

Obstetric — History of serious obstetric complications.

Debility and multiparity (D. & M.) — Extreme debility, characterized by severe anemia, lassitude, progressive deterioration in well being, and depression usually associated with rapid childbearing and large family size. Consideration of the social circumstances was of particular importance in this group.

Other — Eugenic or social circumstances.

For convenience, when the conditions described as medical, psychiatric, or obstetric are being taken together they will be referred to as "medical indications."

Obstetric reasons accounted for 23 of the 24 women having a caesarean section at which sterilization was performed (Table 2). Severe D. & M. were factors in 8 women for whom post-partum sterilization had been recommended but for whom placenta praevia or obstruction necessitated a caesarean section. The remaining woman, a primigravida, had severe heart disease from which she died a few months after the follow-up visit.

TABLE 2.   Indications for Sterilization by Operation Performed

Reason	Caesarean Section and Tubal Ligation	Post-partum Sterilization	Termination and Sterilization	No. of Women
Medical	1	6	15	22
Medical — D. & M.	0	11	1	12
Psychiatric	0	0	2	2
Psychiatric — D. & M.	0	3	2	5
Obstetric	15	1	3	19
Obstetric — D. & M.	8	13	4	25
D. & M.	0	75	17*	92
Other	0	4	5	9
No. of women	24	113	49	186

*Hysterectomy in 3.

In 27 of the 49 women who had a pregnancy terminated in conjunction with sterilization there was a medical indication; D. & M. were additional factors in 7 of these women. Post-partum sterilization had been arranged earlier for some of the remaining 22 women but then postponed for health reasons or because the patient was unwilling to stay in hospital for the extra days required.

102 of the 113 women sterilized in the puerperium or later had extreme debility associated with multiparity. In about a quarter (27 of the 102 women) there was, in addition, a complicating medical factor.

TABLE 3. Per Cent of Women at Sterilization Who Were Aged 35 or Over, Had Four or More Living Children, or Who Were Married to Nonmanual Workers

	Age 35 —	Four or More Children	Husband Nonmanual Worker
Type of operation:			
Caesarean section and tubal ligation	57	37	42
Post-partum sterilization	24	90	8
Termination and sterilization	22	44	12
Indication for sterilization:			
Medical, psychiatric, or obstetric	30	7	32
Medical, psychiatric, or obstetric — D. & M.	33	89	1
D. & M.	24	97	5
Other	11	33	11

Characteristics of sterilized women. Table 3 shows striking differences in women who were sterilized at caesarean section compared with those sterilized after vaginal delivery. In the caesarean-section group women were considerably older, had smaller families, and were of higher socioeconomic status than those sterilized after vaginal delivery. These findings reflect the known incidence of caesarean section; upper-social-class women tend to marry late and the caesarean-section rate is greatly increased in primigravidae over the age of 35 mainly for reasons of uterine dysfunction and fetal distress (Baird 1963).

The women who were sterilized in conjunction with hysterotomy and those who were sterilized post partum were fairly similar in respect of age and husband's socioeconomic group. The women who had a pregnancy terminated had smaller families. This is largely accounted for by the fact that women who have a serious disease are more likely to be sterilized at an earlier stage in childbearing. Table 2 shows that nearly two-and-a-half times as many women who had a pregnancy terminated in conjunction with sterilization, had a serious illness.

The vast majority of women in whom D. & M. were indications for sterilization, had four or more children and with few exceptions they were the wives of manual workers (Table 3). In contrast women sterilized on medical grounds had relatively small families and a third of husbands were in non-manual occupations.

FINDINGS

All 186 women will be considered together, although it is not known how far they are representative of all sterilized women. According to their reactions to sterilization, the women could be divided into three main groups: *(a)* those who regretted being sterilized (8) or who regretted the termination (2), *(b)* those who had no complaint about sterilization but regretted the circumstances that made it necessary (15), and *(c)* those women who were satisfied with sterilization (161).

Regretted sterilization. Eight women regretted having been sterilized. The following case notes will illustrate some of the problems involved in decisions on sterilization and also difficulties of interpretation during follow-up. Details are summarized in Table 4.

TABLE 4. Details of the Women Who Regretted Either Sterilization or Termination

Case no.	Age at Steriliza-tion	Age at Follow-up	Type of Pro-cedure	Reasons for Sterilization	No. of Preg-nancies	No. of Children
Regretted sterilization:						
1	26	35	T.L.	D. & M.	7	4F
2	37	46	H. & S.	PS., D. & M.	8	6
3	33	37	P.P.S.	MED. & M.	13	6
4	37	40	P.P.S.	D. & M.	6	4M
5	34	43	H. & S.	MED.,D.&M.	7	5
6	29	36	P.P.S.	D. & M.	4	4M
7	23	29	H. & S.	MED.	2	1
8	30	34	H. & S.	MED.	3	2
Regretted termination:						
9	33	37	H. & S.	MED.	4	2
10	35	45	H. & S.	D. & M.	4	3

D. & M. = Debility and multiparity.
T.L. = Tubal ligation.
H. & S. = Hysterectomy and sterilization.
PS. = Psychiatric.
MED. = Medical.
F = Female.   M = Male.

CASE 1. A woman sterilized at age twenty-six had been widowed and was contemplating remarriage at the follow-up interview nine years later. She expressed regret that she would be unable to have children by her second husband, but her attitude was partly due to her desire for a son. Four other widows, one of whom was about to remarry, were glad they had been sterilized: they said that otherwise they would probably have had more children and would have found it more difficult to manage. The sixth widow in the series regretted termination, as described below.

CASE 2. This woman regretted that only one of her six children was by her second husband. She thought that a good deal of strife and unhappiness in the family was due to the husband's excessive demands on his only child.

CASE 3. A few months after post partum sterilization this woman's baby died. She regretted not being able to replace it but had made a good adjustment after "a nervous breakdown" treated by her family doctor. (In contrast, a woman who was sterilized after the birth of twins, accepted the death of one of them several months later with equanimity since she had more than she could cope with and had originally wanted the pregnancy terminated.)

CASE 4. This woman had four boys and was obsessional about not having a girl. The circumstances were unusual, since sterilization had been performed after the delivery of a stillborn baby, a girl. Post partum sterilization had been agreed on during pregnancy but was very carefully reconsidered after delivery. The couple were adamant that they did not want more children and insisted on sterilization. Such an example should not set a precedent for postponing sterilization if the baby dies. (Although in this particular case delay might have led to a more satisfactory result, another woman in the series, who had six children, never had any regrets whatsoever at being sterilized the day after her baby's death.)

CASES 5 AND 6. Two motherly women felt "lost" when their youngest child started school and they did not yet have grandchildren to look after. They liked "lots of kiddies around" but they had come too quickly. Both women had additional major medical and social problems in their families and they became exhausted. The woman in Case 6 would have liked a girl and also as a Roman Catholic she felt guilty about being sterilized.

CASE 7. A seriously disabled woman aged twenty-two was carefully nursed through her first pregnancy and labor. She was advised not to have any more children but she conceived a few months later. She blamed her husband entirely and turned against him. She maintained, despite all the medical evidence and opinion, that she would have been able to have more children if the second pregnancy had been delayed. This woman, who cooperated in a longitudinal research project, never adjusted to her life situation. She spent much time in hospital and her mother more or less brought up the child.

CASE 8. A woman reported a vague feeling that "she did wrong to be sterilized." She had no regrets about termination since she only wanted two children. This woman and her husband had considerable experience in contraceptive practice and felt guilty at their failure and the need for surgical intervention. This was an upper-social-class woman in whose social milieu couples usually managed to control their fertility.

Regretted termination. Two women vaguely regretted termination and thought they might have been better to have been sterilized after delivery. One woman (Case 9) could not explain her feelings but she had not wanted more children and at the follow-up interview again said she did not want more. The other woman (Case 10), who had a severely ill husband, thought that termination "was better at the time" and the couple had been insistent in their demands. On his death the altered circumstances and striking reduction in the woman's commitments, coupled with the fact that she was a Roman Catholic, seemed partly to account for her change in attitude. These were two upper-social-class women who, like the one referred to earlier, seemed to feel guilty at not being able to control their fertility and disgraced by the need for termination.

Regretted circumstances that made sterilization necessary. Twelve of the 15 women in this group said that they would have liked more children although three wanted additional children of a particular sex only to get a mixed family. The indications for sterilization had been medical in 11 of the 12 women. Two couples had seriously considered adoption but had decided against it on account of the wife's health. The remaining three women complained of "never feeling well (or right) since sterilization." All had had post-partum sterilization for reasons of extreme debility; two women had six children and the third had five children. A mother who strongly disapproved of sterilization seemed to be a dominant influence in the maladjustment of one of these women, who nevertheless felt that she had enough to do with six children. The woman with five children, a motherly type, thought that she "might like to have another" when her youngest child started school.

Satisfied with sterilization. Of the 161 women who were satisfied, 15 wished that they had been sterilized earlier — since they felt that they had more children than they were able to manage. More women might have felt that they had too many children if they had not delegated permanent responsibility for one or more of their children to relatives (4) or foster parents (3); in addition a mentally defective child was in an institution. Three of the 15 women had had hysterotomy and sterilization and some of the others would have preferred this to post-partum sterilization.

One of four women who expressed regret at not having a mixed family had seven boys. She had had more children than originally intended in the hope of having a girl but felt that she was stretched to the limit with seven children and dared not risk an eighth pregnancy.

Summary of attitudes at follow-up. It is important to consider whether a woman's reaction to sterilization was associated with the type of operation, indication for sterilization, or other factors. First, however, it should be noted that there was no statistically significant difference in the findings of the interviewers.

Table 5 shows that more women were likely to be satisfied if they had had post-partum sterilization (90%). The few women sterilized for eugenic or social reasons were entirely satisfied. The results were least satisfactory when sterilization had been performed on medical grounds alone, since a quarter of these women would have liked more children.

Table 5 shows a striking association between satisfaction and increasing family size. Most workers have reported similar findings. Ekblad (1961) considered that the possession of even one child considerably diminished the risk of regret. Nevertheless the only childless woman in the Aberdeen series was entirely satisfied; she had been sterilized when her third pregnancy

TABLE 5. Attitudes of Women at Follow-up in Relation to Type of Operation and Other Factors

	Regretted Sterilization or Termination	Regretted Circumstances of Sterilization	Satisfied	Total
Type of operation:				
Tubal ligation with caesarean section	0	4	20 *(83%)*	24
Post-partum sterilization	4	7	102 *(90%)*	113
Termination and sterilization	6	4	39 *(79%)*	49
Indications for sterilization:				
Medical, psychiatric, or obstetric	3	10	29 *(69%)*	42
Medical, psychiatric, obstetric — D. & M.	3	1	39 *(91%)*	43
D. & M.	4	4	84 *(91%)*	92
Other	0	0	9 *(100%)*	9
No. of children:				
<2	3	7	20 *(66%)*	30
3	2	4	18 *(75%)*	24
4	2	1	41 *(93%)*	44
>5	3	3	82 *(93%)*	88
Age and sterilization:				
<30 yr.	3	6	64 *(87%)*	73
30-34 yr.	4	6	52 *(84%)*	62
>35 yr.	3	3	45 *(88%)*	51
Husband's occupation:				
Non-manual	3	4	18 *(72%)*	25
Skilled manual	3	4	59 *(89%)*	66
Other manual	4	7	84 *(88%)*	95
Total	10 *(5%)*	15 *(8%)*	161 *(87%)*	186

was terminated, primarily for psychiatric reasons, but there were complicating obstetric, eugenic, and social factors. It is interesting to note the high proportion of women with four or more children who were satisfied with sterilization (93%) since another study in Aberdeen showed that in the 1950s most women wanted two or three children and none wanted more than four (Thompson and Illsley, 1968).

Age at sterilization seems to be relatively unimportant in determining reactions. Many workers elsewhere have reported unfavorable results in younger women and a minimum age of thirty is sometimes suggested (Naville, 1952; Boulware et al., 1954; Adams, 1964).

Table 5 also shows similarity of reaction among wives of skilled manual and other manual workers (88% satisfied, 4% regretted being sterilized). The inclusion of the two women who regretted termination largely accounts for the less satisfactory findings in the wives of nonmanual workers (72% satisfied, 5% regretted being sterilized, and 10% regretted termination).

Attitude to coitus. A major concern of couples contemplating sterilization is the likely effect on coitus. Although the information is obviously very superficial, at the follow-up interviews the women reported on their sexual relations after sterilization as follows: improved 81, unchanged 75, deteriorated 21, uncertain 9.

Improvement was usually attributed to the freedom from fear of conception and greater ability to relax. The women no longer tried to avoid intercourse, there was less quarreling, and the marital relationship was happier; indeed several women thought that sterilization had saved the marriage. A few said that for the first time they sometimes took the initiative in sexual activity or that they had experienced orgasm only since sterilization.

Some of the women who said that their attitude was unchanged added that they had never been very interested in coitus nor did they find it pleasurable; sterilization had made no difference in this respect.

One of the women who reported a deterioration blamed this on the fact that she had had a hysterectomy; she felt that coitus would probably not have deteriorated if she had had tubal ligation. Twenty per cent of the women who regretted the circumstances of sterilization reported a deterioration in their attitude to coitus, compared with 10% in the other two groups.

Woodside (1949) in her follow-up of mentally normal married women who had been sterilized in North Carolina, found that the few women who reported adverse results in sexual relations presented symptoms of a neurotic personality and poor emotional adjustment even before sterilization. Black and Sclare (1968), from Glasgow, concluded that sterilization has little influence on basic psychiatric problems. No psychiatric interpretation of the Aberdeen findings has been attempted.

The follow-up studies produced no evidence that husbands were driven to seek extramarital relationships as a consequence of the wife being sterilized, although some women reported a very difficult period of adjustment directly after the operation.

At least five husbands were known to have indulged in extramarital relationships before the wife was sterilized and they did not change their habits. Two women had had illegitimate children born since marriage; the husbands had spent long periods in hospital and prison, respectively. Two couples separated, two and six years after sterilization, respectively; both marriages had always been unhappy as the husbands seldom worked, they gambled and drank, and one had a prison record.

It is sometimes said that sterilization will encourage promiscuity in the woman. A husband, interviewed independently, confirmed that his wife associated with other men. He felt that sterilization was at least partly responsible for her behavior which included loss of interest in the house and their six children. There was a striking increase in the wife's interest in coitus after sterilization but the husband was not very interested. He was a steady worker and more home-loving than his wife. She had complained both before and after sterilization of her boredom with domesticity and of her "unexciting" husband. The evidence is inconclusive on whether she had had extramarital intercourse before sterilization or not.

Health. The gynecological history since sterilization was obtained for 121 women who were visited at home. Three women had become pregnant three to nine years later and been readmitted for further operation. Forty-four women attributed a variety of gynecological conditions to sterilization.

It is difficult to assess the significance of some of the complaints: a few women who complained said that they had had little experience of menstruation before sterilization, since they had been in an almost continuous state of pregnancy or post-partum amenorrhoea since the menarche, some said that they accepted irregular and heavy periods or dysmenorrhoea as a natural consequence of sterilization, a disadvantage far outweighed by the advantages it conferred, others were prepared to suffer pain and inconvenience rather than risk having a hysterectomy, an operation greatly feared, particularly by women in the lower social classes who frequently lack knowledge and understanding of female anatomy and of the physiology of reproduction.

It is likely that women with the most severe or prolonged gynecological conditions will ultimately be seen by a gynecologist. An opportunity was taken, therefore, in the course of another research project, to examine the histories of 55 sterilized women who attended the gynecological clinic in one year. The association of the gynecological complaint with the sterilization operation was certain in five (four failed sterilization), possible in three (symptoms were mild and laparotomy was not performed), and unlikely in the remaining 47. Of these 47 women, two had cancer of cervix, 22 had menorrhagia, 16 had vaginal discharge, and 7 miscellaneous disorders usually of a minor nature. All the evidence available indicated that sterilization was unrelated to the majority of postoperative gynecological complaints. Black and Sclare (1968) reported similar findings. More women among those who regretted either being sterilized or the necessity for sterilization reported adverse effects on menstruation and/or on coitus than did those who were satisfied, but the differences between the groups were not statistically significant.

Chronic disease, mental illness, poor physique, or extreme debility manifested by lethargy, anemia, and depression were frequent in all groups. Some women required prolonged convalescence after the operation. The debilitated women with large families frequently said that it took about two years before they felt the full benefit in general health. The improvement in the physical and mental health of some women was so great that they were almost unrecognizable by the medical social worker who had known them before. Serious progressive disease resulted in a deterioration in the condition of some women. The onset of menopausal changes in the older women complicates the assessment of the state of health and well being.

Few women attributed variations in weight to sterilization. The woman's own comments on weight change are available for 85 women in series A, B, and D. A striking increase, up to about 3 stones (20 kg.), was reported by 46 women, and only 14 said that they had lost weight since being sterilized; the weight had remained constant in 19 women and had fluctuated in 6. The women thought that gain in weight was due to age (menopause), "sitting around and eating more," stopping smoking, or the result of other operations such as thyroidectomy. Several women were having treatment for obesity, whereas others said that they were merely regaining weight lost in early marriage. The women attributed weight loss to "nerves," gastric ulcers, metabolic disturbances, and severe gynecological disorders.

DISCUSSION

Great variation in the circumstances of the women and their families makes comparisons and assessment difficult. Serious health problems, social situations, or association with a termination of pregnancy complicate interpretation of a woman's reaction to sterilization. Further, in this follow-up, there was no control group of unsterilized women nor was the interval between sterilization and subsequent interview standardized.

In general, one can say that sterilization had conferred great practical and psychological benefits, such as better health, removal of the fear of pregnancy, and improvement in marital and family relationships. The vast majority of the women in the follow-up series were satisfied and were enthusiastic advocates of sterilization.

Where the result was unsatisfactory there was usually an explanation to be found, for example, previous history of an unsatisfactory personality, which, as Woodside (1949) pointed out, is not changed by sterilization, or unsatisfied maternal feeling (Ekblad, 1961), or changed circumstances. The findings suggest that women may be upset by the disapproval of their church. Also upper-class women may have a sense of failure in being sterilized since fertility is usually controlled by contraception in their social group.

Other workers agree that sterilization is most successful in mothers of large families as a final measure of limiting family size. In some Aberdeen women, it would have been more constructive and beneficial if undertaken earlier.

Before sterilization is undertaken, every aspect of a woman's health, marriage, and family life needs to be considered. This has been possible in Aberdeen because the medical services are coordinated and the personnel involved in collecting the necessary information on which the decision is based are integrated. With careful selection of women and sympathetic care, the results of sterilization have been most satisfactory. Since most upper-social-class couples manage to control their fertility, sterilization is seldom necessary in women in this class, except in cases of severe disability or after repeated caesarean section. By contrast, in the lower social classes, it has been freely used and is widely accepted. Mothers encourage daughters, and friends advise neighbors to have their "tubes tied" as a "relief from the tyranny of excessive fertility" (Baird, 1965).

The future need for sterilization may be lessened, as more acceptable and efficient methods of contraception become available. Oral contraceptives are now being used by large numbers of women in all social classes. The idea of the intrauterine device is attractive to many women but its advantages are offset by a high failure rate and medical complications. These methods were not available to the women in our follow-up series. They will undoubtedly reduce substantially in all social classes the number of unplanned and unwanted babies. Nevertheless, tubal ligation may remain the most satisfactory solution for some women who want to finish childbearing early and who may not be able or willing to use other contraceptive methods. In certain circumstances vasectomy in the husband may prove to be an acceptable alternative; the demand for this relatively simple operation and its results are being investigated by the Simon Population Trust (1967).

We thank Miss J. Aitken-Swan, Dr. J. E. Macgregor, and Miss M. D. Campbell who interviewed women in groups D & E *(a)* & *(b),* respectively, and Prof. I. MacGillivray, Prof. R. Illsley and other colleagues for their help in the preparation of this paper.

REFERENCES
Adams, T. W. (1964) *Am. J. Obstet. Gynec.* 89, 395.
Baird, D. (1963) *J. Obstet. Gynaec.* 70, 204.
—— (1965) *Br. med. J.* ii, 1141.
Black, W. P., Sclare, A. B. (1968) *J. Obstet. Gynaec. Br. Commonw.* 75, 219.
Boulware, T. M., Howe, C. D., Simpson, S. T. (1954) *Am. J. Obstet. Gynec.* 68, 1124.
Ekblad, M. (1961) *Acta psychiat. scand.* suppl. no. 161.
Naville, A. (1952) *Praxis,* 41, 1020.
Simon Population Trust (1967) Family Planning 16, 72.
Thompson, B., Illsley, R. (1968) Unpublished.
Woodside, M. (1949) *West. J. Surg.* 57, 600.

2   STERILIZATION BY TUBAL LIGATION — A FOLLOW-UP STUDY

by W. P. Black, M.D., and A. B. Sclare

Indications for sterilization may be broadly divided into three groups — medical, eugenic, and socio-economic. Medical indications are generally acceptable and can be evaluated in terms of the subsequent physical and mental welfare of the patient. Eugenic indications, although capable of some statistical assessment, are relatively uncommon and their final analysis frequently depends on complex psychosocial factors. The socio-economic group, in which the main indication is multiparity, is the largest and most complex because the operation is permissive, being performed at the request of the patient and her husband and with consideration of prevailing ethical views.

It would be easy for doctors to limit indications for sterilization to those which are strictly medical, as they are medical men and not socio-economic prophets. Socio-economic indications, however, should not be based on sentimental guesses but on facts derived from general medical practice and family planning experience. Unwillingness to sterilize a patient may stem from religious conviction, fear of litigation, or doubt about the medical value of the operation. The operation should contribute to the patient's physical and mental well being and have no detrimental effects. The risks of the operation need to be weighed against the possible effects of further childbearing on the patient's health, social well being, marriage and family life, bearing in mind her age, parity, and religion.

CLINICAL MATERIAL

This paper presents data about 480 patients who were sterilized by tubal ligation in Glasgow Royal Infirmary and Eastern District Hospital from January 1961 to July 1966, and reports the results of a gynecological and psychiatric assessment of 168 (45 per cent) of these patients who were examined one to five years later.

A modification of the Pomeroy method was performed by crushing a loop of Fallopian tube, doubly ligating it and excising the loop. The operation was undertaken with the written consent of the patient and her husband after full explanation of what was involved. Sterilization is like any other operation in that the law can neither compel a surgeon to perform it, nor punish him for performing it, provided that he exercises his judgment in good faith, keeps to the dictates of his conscience, and that the indications are those that are generally accepted.

The following information was extracted from the case records. Eighty sterilizations were carried out at the time of caesarean section (Section Group), 200 were performed within a few days of delivery (Postpartum Group), and 200 three months or more after confinement (Interval Group). There was no record of a pregnancy following sterilization.

The proportion of Roman Catholics (32.7 per cent) was similar to that of the general population surrounding the hospitals (33.5 per cent) noted by Smith and Sclare (1964) (Table 1). The ages and parity distribution (Tables 2 and 3) were similar in the Interval and Postpartum Groups with the peak

TABLE 1   Time of Sterilization and Religion of Patients

	At Caesarean Section	Within a Few Days of Delivery	Three or More Months After Delivery
Roman Catholic	29	71	57
Other denominations	51	129	143
Total	80	200	200

TABLE 2   Ages of Patients Sterilized

Age	Sterilized at Caesarean Section	Sterilized at Other Times
Under 25 years	11	14
25-29 years	22	92
30-34 years	23	164
35-39 years	17	100
Over 39 years	7	30
Total	80	400

TABLE 3   Parity of Patients Sterilized

Parity	Sterilized at Caesarean Section	Sterilized at Other Times
1-4	55	85
5-8	18	252
Over 8	7	63
Total	80	400

TABLE 4   Indications for Sterilization

Indications	Sterilized at Caesarean Section	Sterilized at Other Times
Multiparity	15	299
Previous Caesarean section	40	4
Medical reasons	25	97
Cardiac disease	2	25
Bad obstetric history	8	20
Rhesus disease	9	6
Psychiatric disorder	–	10
Other conditions	6	36

age at 30-34 years and the peak parity at 5 to 8. The sterilizations performed at the time of caesarean section were, as
expected, in younger patients of lower parity.

INDICATIONS

The indications for sterilization were divided into three
groups — multiparity (5 or more children), previous caesarean
section and medical reasons (Table 4). It will be seen that
psychiatric reasons were infrequent. In the operation performed
at the time of caesarean section the commonest reason was
previous section; 80 per cent of the sterilizations for this indication were performed at the time of the second section. In the
other cases, whether the operation was performed in the
puerperium or later, multiparity was the commonest indication.

POSTOPERATIVE COMPLICATIONS

Postoperative complications were most frequent in the
patients sterilized at the time of caesarean section (Table 5).
Pyrexia (99.4° F.) was noted in 29 per cent of cases and was
notifiable (100.4° F.) in 10 per cent. Morbidity following
caesarean section, however, was not increased by concurrent
sterilization. One patient who had a caesarean section because
of concealed accidental hemorrhage had a pulmonary embolism
two weeks after the operation and subsequently died.

TABLE 5   Postoperative Complications

Complication	At Caesarean Section	Within a Few Days of Delivery	Three or More Months After Delivery
None	48	155	186
Pyrexia (99.4° F.)	23	17	13
Infection of chest	10	11	5
Infection of wound	6	22	6
Infection of renal tract	4	1	5
Thrombophlebitis	2	2	—
Thromboembolism	1	1	—
Mild ileus	3	—	—

Time of Sterilization

Complications were less frequent in the Interval than in the Postpartum Group in which there were more minor complications. The average stay in hospital after sterilization was similar for both groups. Postoperative complications were not related to the indication for sterilization. The majority of postpartum sterilizations were performed on the second or third postnatal day and the incidence of complications was not affected by the day of operation. Postpartum patients who had an obstetric operation under general anesthesia before sterilization showed an increased incidence of complications. Six of the 8 patients in the group (three cases of breech extraction, three cases of forceps delivery, two cases of manual removal of placenta) experienced complications after sterilization. One of these patients developed a pulmonary embolism from which she recovered. Complications were not increased in the 33 patients in the Interval Group in whom sterilization was accompanied by additional surgical procedures (ovarian resection, curettage, appendectomy, ovarian cystectomy, salpingo-oöphorectomy, repair of umbilical hernia, vaginal plastic repair). In all, 264 patients from the three groups came for examination six weeks after operation when the only abnormalities detected were 11 minor problems with wound healing.

GYNECOLOGICAL FOLLOW-UP ASSESSMENT

The gynecological assessment of the 168 patients followed up comprised a full gynecological history, pelvic examination and cervical cytology. This sample of 168 patients was statistically comparable with the total 480 patients in all the aspects previously detailed. Twenty-eight (17 per cent) of them required gynecological treatment; 19 had chronic cervicitis; 6 complained of menstrual upset necessitating diagnostic curettage; two were shown to have preinvasive carcinoma of cervix; one patient underwent ovarian cystectomy. None of these conditions could be associated in any way with the operation of sterilization.

PSYCHIATRIC FOLLOW-UP ASSESSMENT

A standard interview was carried out with each patient followed up and details of any psychiatric disorder prior to sterilization were retrospectively determined; the nature and treatment of any such illness were noted and the patient's personality and background explored. Enquiries were made about (1) mental status, (2) marital adjustment, (3) psychosexual adjustment, and (4) economic adjustment. For each factor comparison was made between the patient's condition immediately before operation and that at the time of examination. The patient's own views and attitudes were also assessed when classifying the shift in each category as "better," "same," or "worse."

The trend was towards improvement in all four psychosocial functions after sterilization (Table 6). These findings

TABLE 6   Psychosocial Function After Sterilization

	Mental Status	Marital Adjustment	Psychosexual Adjustment	Economic Adjustment
Better	99 (59%)	89 (53%)	45 (27%)	82 (49%)
Same	45 (27%)	68 (40%)	108 (64%)	84 (50%)
Worse	24 (4%)	11 (7%)	15 (9%)	2 (1%)
Total	168	168	168	168

were not related to the indications for sterilization. The psychological benefits of sterilization were vividly described by many
patients, e.g., "I have a great sense of relief now," "I don't
have to worry about having children now." Many described
new-found satisfaction in the marriage relationship, and a considerable number commenced part-time employment after the
operation, thus broadening their horizons and improving their
economic situation.

Careful history taking at the time of the study disclosed
retrospectively that 37 patients (22 per cent) had definite
evidence of psychiatric disorder before being sterilized; they
described emotional disturbances which necessitated
attendance upon the family doctor or psychiatrist. It should
be made clear, however, that there was a psychiatric indication for sterilization in only two patients in the follow-up
sample. The 37 patients with "antecedent psychiatric disorder"
were classified as follows: psychoneurosis, 30; psychosis, 2;
personality disorder, 3; and mental subnormality, 2. When these
37 patients were compared with the other 131 patients it was
found that in respect of mental status, marital adjustment,
and psychosexual adjustment, those with antecedent psychiatric
disorder benefited less than the others from sterilization.

Deteriorations in adjustment occurred in 39 patients.
Analysis of these 39 patients revealed that they could be
grouped as follows: antecedent psychiatric disorder, 18;
extraneous postoperative circumstances, 15; postoperative regret
or guilt, 6. "Extraneous postoperative circumstances" included
important events such as family disruption, bereavement,
serious nongynecological disorder, etc., which were unrelated
to the sterilization. There was no difference in the age distribution, in the proportion of Roman Catholics, in the timing
of the operation, nor in the frequencies of the different indications for operation between the 39 patients with deterioration
in adjustment and the other 129 patients. Nor did the "regret-
guilt" group differ from the total sample in these respects and
only one patient in the "regret-guilt" group was under 30 years
of age.

DISCUSSION

The indications for sterilization, viz. multiparity (65.4 per cent), which was often associated with socio-economic factors, medical reasons (25.4 per cent), and previous caesarean section (9.2 per cent) are similar to those reported by Adams (1964) and reflect the current trend towards a more liberal approach to the socio-economic group.

In this series of patients complications were infrequent and mostly of a minor nature. One patient, however, died of pulmonary embolism after caesarean section for an obstetric complication, and another patient developed pulmonary embolism after sterilization in the puerperium after forceps delivery under general anesthesia.

Postoperative complications were not related to the age or parity of the patient nor to the indication for sterilization. The postpartum day of operation did not influence the incidence of complications but the Postpartum Group of patients experienced more complications than those in the Interval Group. This was particularly noticeable in those patients who had an obstetric operation under general anesthesia prior to sterilization in the puerperium and suggests that such patients would be better served by interval sterilization. White (1966) found that the interval procedure provided the lowest complication rate in his series. Steptoe (1967) has described a laparoscopic technique for sterilization which is not applicable to puerperal patients but which requires only 48 hours' stay in hospital, and this may be the method of choice in the future.

Neither the postoperative examination at six weeks after operation nor follow-up examination more than one year afterwards disclosed any important physical ill effects from the procedure. The incidental gynecological problems at late follow-up examination were those to be expected in patients of this age and parity, and there was no evidence that sterilization was followed by an increased incidence of gynecological problems such as menstrual upsets.

The psychiatric follow-up revealed that sterilization was generally associated with improvement in the mental, marital, and economic adjustment of the patients. The patients were freed from fear of future pregnancy and showed diminished tension and irritability within the marriage relationship and increased ability to control their economic situation. The improvement in their psychosexual adjustment, however, was comparatively slight. This finding is in keeping with that of Ekblad (1961), and possibly indicates that fear of conception is not a major factor in explaining poor sexual adjustment.

When the patients were classified according to the presence or absence of psychiatric disorder before sterilization, it was found that the 37 patients (22 per cent) who were psychiatrically disturbed before sterilization showed less benefit in their mental, marital, and psychosexual adjustment afterwards than the remaining 131 patients. Ekblad (1961) similarly found that 31 per cent of his patients suffered from chronic neurosis although, as in this present series, this was not the actual indication for sterilization.

Chronic environmental stress no doubt explains the common occurrence of neurotic problems in multiparous women in the lower socio-economic groups. The results indicate that all candidates for sterilization should have their mental as well as their physical state assessed before operation. If there is a clear history of chronic psychoneurosis there is likely to be less improvement in psychosocial functioning after sterilization. Sterilization can be expected to improve socio-economic functioning but has little influence on any basic psychiatric problems.

The 39 patients who accounted for the deteriorations in adjustment could readily be classified in terms of antecedent psychiatric disorder (18 patients), extraneous postoperative circumstance (15 patients), and postoperative regret or guilt (6 patients). The patients in whom extraneous stresses occurred after sterilization may well have fared better in the absence of such circumstances. The six patients with regret-guilt (3.6 per cent of the sample), however, arouse most concern about the selection of patients for sterilization. This group could not be differentiated from the rest of the sample. Norris (1964) noted that his dissatisfied patients (9.1 per cent of his series) tended to be Roman Catholic, in the lower socio-economic groups and under the age of 30 years. Ekblad (1961) found that the 7 per cent of his patients who later regretted the operation tended to have unstable marriages. Such correlations did not emerge in the present study. Adams (1964) advocated a "cooling-off" period of at least 30 days between making the decision to carry out sterilization and the actual operation, in order to minimize subsequent regret. While this would appear to be sound advice, the present findings do not support his view that immediate sterilization, e.g., at the time of caesarean section, is associated with regret.

It may well be that since a patient's final decision to surrender her reproductive potential involves complex and ambiguous emotions, a small residue of discontented individuals can be expected even among a group of patients selected for sterilization with the greatest discrimination. The finality of sterilization by tubal ligation by the Pomeroy technique has to be accepted when a decision is made, and should the operation be performed on medical grounds, the permanence of the method is an obvious advantage. When the operation is performed for socio-economic reasons it is possible that a patient may have future regrets and even wish the procedure undone. Because this is more likely to occur in younger women, and since reversal of this type of sterilization is seldom achieved, it should not be freely advocated for younger patients, particularly if they are of low parity or have a chronic neurosis.

SUMMARY
Data about 480 patients sterilized at the time of caesarean section, in the early puerperium, or subsequently, have been presented. The results of a gynecological and psychiatric assessment one to five years after sterilization on 168 of these patients are discussed. If a patient requires sterilization and has had an obstetric operation requiring a general anesthetic, the sterilization should be performed after the puerperium. Significant ill effects directly attributable to the operation were not apparent at follow-up examination one or more years after sterilization. An improvement in social and mental well being was found in 96.4 per cent of the patients although those who had a chronic neurosis experienced less benefit. A small

group (3.6 per cent) of patients at late follow-up manifested regret or guilt about their sterilization.

3 MEDICAL AND PSYCHOLOGICAL SEQUELAE OF SURGICAL STERILIZATION OF WOMEN

by Manuel E. Paniagua, M.D., Matthew Tayback, José L. Janer, and José L. Vázquez

From the Family Planning Association of Puerto Rico, the Johns Hopkins School of Hygiene, and the Department of Public Health and Preventive Medicine, University of Puerto Rico.

This study was made possible by a grant from the Population Council.

When fertility control is considered a prime family objective for social stability and economic advancement and when nonsurgical techniques of contraception prove difficult to use, surgical sterilization of the woman would appear to be a rational alternative. However, it is reasonable to demand information on the medical and psychological sequelae of sterilization of women before the acceptance of this procedure as a justifiable medical action. This paper is concerned with the presentation of such data: it was obtained from a systematic follow-up of women, residents of Puerto Rico, who were sterilized on their request and with the consent of their husbands. With few exceptions, the sterilizations were requested to limit the size of family for social and economic reasons rather than medical reasons.

A review of the literature pertaining to tubal ligation (3) indicates that many of the papers are concerned with studies of the outcome of sterilization performed for medical reasons and cover operations undertaken before the advent of modern antibiotics and chemotherapy. Consequently, information reported on death, morbidity, or psychological sequelae may not be relevant to a series of patients in whom the primary consideration for sterilization was social or economic necessity and who were operated upon with benefit of antibiotics or chemotherapeutic agents to minimize infection.

It would appear, then, that earlier studies of the risk of death associated with puerperal tubal sterilization provide estimates of mortality risk ranging from 3.0 per 1,000 to .3 per 1,000 with the likelihood that the higher risk is associated with operations undertaken for impelling medical reasons, while the lower risk is associated with operations on women seeking control of fertility for social or economic circumstances.

PSYCHOLOGICAL SEQUELAE

If the mortality risk associated with sterilization in women proves to be of tolerable dimensions, there could still be substantial reservation concerning the use of this procedure if serious disability or dissatisfaction were to result as a consequence of emotional changes induced by the operation. A large number of studies on this issue are found in the literature including contributions from European and Indian authors (7-9). The difficulty in reaching meaningful conclusions from these investigations derives from the differences between the characteristics of one patient group and those of another. Barnes and Zuspan (10) in a careful follow-up study, secured responses to 40 different questions by interviews conducted by a social worker in the patient's home. For 311 women, of an originally selected series of 457, successful interviews were completed. The principal findings were that 90 per cent of patients who had taken the initiative to request sterilization expressed no subsequent regret, while among women who had been persuaded to undergo sterilization, 69 per cent had no regret, 27 per cent were ambivalent, and 5 per cent had definite regret. In this connection, it was found that where the indication for sterilization was multiparity, the proportion expressing no regret was 92 per cent. It is safe to infer that, by and large, in instances of multiparity the patients themselves take the initiative in seeking sterilization.

STUDY DESIGN

Since 1956, the Family Planning Association of Puerto Rico, a private, nonprofit organization devoted to orientation, research, and direct services in the field of population control, has been giving advice and economic assistance to people de-

siring to terminate their reproductive capacity by means of surgical sterilization. Such help is given only on request. The bene-
ficiaries must meet certain requirements set by the Medical
Committee of the Association when the operation is requested
for economic reasons. These standards are as follows: minimum
age of 20 for women and 25 for men; at least 3 living children;
emotional stability; a thorough understanding of the irreversi-
bility of the procedure; and reasonable expectance of permanence of the union. In addition, couples are advised to give the
matter serious thought and consideration. When there is some
medical or social indication for sterilization, the cases are
evaluated individually and some or all of the rules may be waived.

Early in the planning of the study it was decided that
the number of completed interviews should be at least 10 per
cent of the total operations performed and that the best method
for obtaining reliable information was the personal interview
conducted in the home of the patient by a person profession-
ally trained for this type of work.

Characteristics of the sample. The median age of the 519
patients who underwent sterilization in the sample studied was
30.1 years with 70 per cent of them falling within the age interval of 25 to 34 years. Fifteen per cent reported ages under 25
years.

Their spouses had a median age of 35.2 years, and 74.7
per cent reported ages between 25 and 44 years. Only 3.9 per
cent reported ages under 25 years, while 17.5 per cent were reported to be age 45 years and over.

The educational attainments of both the patients and
their respective spouses were essentially the same as those reported in the 1960 Census of Puerto Rico for the population
aged 25 years or more, namely 4.3 for women and 4.8 for men.
The median number of completed school years was found to
be 4.2 for the patients and 4.5 for their spouses. Of the 519 patients, only 28, or 5.4 per cent, reported the completion of 12 or
more years of schooling. Of these 28 patients, only four had
had some schooling beyond the twelfth grade.

As could be expected in a country predominantly Catholic by tradition, 440 or 84.8 per cent of the patients reported

TABLE 1. Sterilization of Women Performed
under the Auspices of the Family Planning
Association of Puerto Rico, 1956 through 1961

Year	Operation (No.)	Patients Interviewed (No.)	Patients Interviewed in Corresponding Year (%)
1956	284	45	15.8
1957	427	85	19.9
1958	524	68	13.0
1959	733	93	12.7
1960	779	144	18.5
1961	643	84	13.1
Total	3,390	519	15.3

Roman Catholicism as their religion. This is somewhat larger than the estimated percentage of Catholics among the general population. Protestant groups were represented by 58 or 11.2 per cent of the patients. Of the remaining 21 patients, 3 belonged to other religious groups and 18 belonged to no organized religion.

Roman Catholicism was also predominant among the spouses, as it was found to be the religion of 399 or 76.9 per cent. However, 55 or 10.6 per cent were nonbelievers, a substantially larger proportion than that found among the patients, or female group. Of the remaining 65 patients, 45 belonged to Protestant groups, 7 to other groups, and 13 did not state their religion.

With respect to attendance at religious services the 519 patients reported as follows:

	Patients	%
Attended regularly	123	23.7
Attended sometimes only	309	59.5
Never attended (includes the 18 who do not belong to any religion)	87	16.8
Total	519	100.0

Among the 440 Catholic patients, regular attendance at religious services was reported by 21.4 per cent.

At the date of operation the number of marital unions which the patients reported was as follows:

No. of Unions	No. of Patients	%
1	366	70.5
2	116	22.3
3+	29	5.6
Not stated or no union	8	1.6
Total	519	100.0

The median number of children for the 519 patients at the time of the operation was found to be 3.7. Those with 3 or more children amounted to 475 or 91.5 per cent of the whole group, while those with 5 or more were 222 or 42.8 per cent.

Only 262 or 51.5 per cent of all the patients reported the use of some method of birth control prior to sterilization. Of these, 148, or 26.6 per cent, of all the 519 patients reported the regular use of such methods.

Table 2 presents the number of patients reporting the use of each specified method.

Attention is called to the small number of patients reporting the use of rhythm or coitus interruptus.

TABLE 2

Method	No. of Users	Per Cent of 262 Users	Per Cent of 519 Patients
Condom	82	31.3	15.8
Jelly	76	29.0	14.6
Foam tablets	42	16.0	8.1
Diaphragm	35	13.4	6.7
Coitus interruptus	4	1.5	0.8
Rhythm	4	1.5	0.8
Other methods	73	27.9	14.1
Not stated	4	1.5	0.8

TABLE 3

Reason for Preferring Operation	No.	%
Safer method	208	54.9
Objection to other methods	134	35.4
Medical reasons	35	9.2
Not stated	2	0.5
Total	379	100.0

Of the 257 patients who said they had not used any birth control method prior to sterilization, 170, or 61.1 per cent, reported knowing about one or more methods.

When asked about the reasons for having preferred the operation to the use of other birth control methods, 379, or 73.0 per cent of the 519 patients, gave a single reason for their preference, while 140 or 27.0 per cent expressed more than one. The 379 patients who gave a single reason for having preferred the operation were distributed as shown in Table 3.

Of the remaining 140 patients who gave more than one reason for having preferred the operation, 105 mentioned the safeness of the method as one of the reasons for their preference. This means that "safeness of the method" was reported by 313, or 60.3 per cent, of all the 519 patients.

In 441, or 85 per cent, of the cases the spouse decidedly approved the operation, while in only 19, or 3.9 per cent, he decidedly opposed it. In the remaining 59 cases the spouse approved the operation but with some reservations. Opposition on religious grounds amounted to only 9, or 1.7 per cent, of the cases.

Opposition from close relatives other than the spouse was also very small. In 495, or 95.9 per cent, of the cases close relatives decidedly approved the operation. Opposition on religious grounds from close relatives was observed again in only 9, or 1.7 per cent, of the cases.

When asked about what made them decide on the operation, the patients responded as shown in Table 4.

TABLE 4

Reason	No.	%
Economic	232	44.7
Poor health	92	17.7
Social	14	2.7
Economic and health	102	19.7
Economic and social	40	7.7
Social and health	7	1.3
Social, economic, and health	8	1.6
Other	24	4.6
Total	519	100.0

Economic reasons were thus involved in 73.7 per cent of the replies, while health reasons were involved in 40.3 per cent and social ones in 13.3 per cent.

MEDICAL SEQUELAE

Mortality rate. No deaths have occurred in the immediate postoperative period in 5,716 women sterilized under the auspices of the Family Planning Association of Puerto Rico from July, 1956, to December, 1962. Though this is a selected and screened group, the absence of fatalities is highly significant and has been critically questioned by several investigators including ourselves. In an effort to clarify this point we have attacked it from two different angles.

A careful survey of the records of several private and government hospitals was made (Table 5) and again no deaths were found.

TABLE 5

Hospital	Type	Period Covered	No. Operations
1	Private	1952-1960	1,972
2	Private	1952-1961	611
3	Government	1950-1960	2,002
4	Government	1951-1961	921
5	Government	1951-1960	1,127
Total			6,633

Another survey was conducted in collaboration with the Bureau of Vital Statistics of the Department of Health of The Commonwealth of Puerto Rico in which death certificates of all women between the ages of 20 and 45 who had died during 1960 were scrutinized and again no evidence was found where the death could be directly related to the operation. Not all these certificates are completely reliable because many of them are filled out by physicians who never took care of the deceased or even knew her. We believe there must be some cases in which sterilization is, at least indirectly, related to death, but, again, this would not show in the death certificate.

As an example, there is the case of M. F. F., a 31-year-old woman who was sterilized in the Municipal Hospital of a small town and next day went into shock which did not respond to usual treatment. She was transferred to a larger District Hospital where she was reoperated upon and died 2 days later. The death certificate lists shock caused by hemorrhagic infarction of small bowel as the immediate cause of death. The preceding operation is not mentioned.

MORBIDITY

Immediate complications. Among the 519 women included in this series, there were 21 cases of wound infection (4 per cent) and 6 of hemorrhage (1.2 per cent) plus 10 other minor complications. Four hundred seventy-nine women (92.3 per cent) reported no immediate postoperative complications.

TABLE 6.   Changes in Overall Health

Changes	Objective Evaluation		Subjective Evaluation	
	No.	%	No.	%
Better	219	42.2	216	41.6
Same	207	39.9	224	43.2
Worse	93	17.9	79	15.2
Total	519	100.0	519	100.0

Late sequelae. It is obviously very difficult to evaluate retrospectively a variety of symptoms and determine whether they are in any way related to a previous operation. In our questionnaire we attempted to break them down into specific complaints, determine whether they were present prior to operation and, if so, whether there had been any change in the character, duration, severity, etc. General and specific questions were asked from different angles and each woman was requested to evaluate subjectively any changes in her general health. A comparison of postoperative changes in health as evaluated objectively by us from the answers to several different questions, and subjectively by the women themselves, is shown in Table 6.

We were agreeably surprised by the high degree of correlation found. It is noteworthy that between 15 and 18 per cent of the women were apparently in worse health than previously, although after studying individual records it is apparent that many of the reported changes in health had nothing to do with the operation.

PSYCHOLOGIC SEQUELAE

The emotional consequences of sterilization were studied by inquiring in detail about changes in sexual relations (including libido, frequency of coitus, and frequency of orgasm); changes in personal relations with the husband and changes in social relations with the rest of the family and with the community; and general satisfaction with the results of the operation.

Changes in several parameters of sexual relationships are presented in Figure 1. For each of these variables the pattern appears to be relatively constant. Close to 60 per cent of respondents indicate no change. About 12 per cent report an increase in sexual activity while about 24 per cent report a decline.

Further confirmation that sexual relations are substantially unaffected following sterilization is gained from consideration of data describing change in frequency of orgasm as reported by the patient on interview. This information is shown in Table 7.

TABLE 7. Changes in Frequency of Orgasm After Operation

Changes in Frequency of Orgasm	No. Patients	Per Cent Total
More frequent	54	10.4
Same as before	335	64.5
Less frequent	90	17.3
Not stated	40	7.7
Total	519	99.9

About 2 of 3 women who were sterilized stated that there was no change in the frequency of orgasm following operation. Because of the extreme emotional tone associated with this experience, accuracy of recall of such information is very high.

The changes in personal relations with the spouse and with the rest of the family and the community are shown in Table 8.

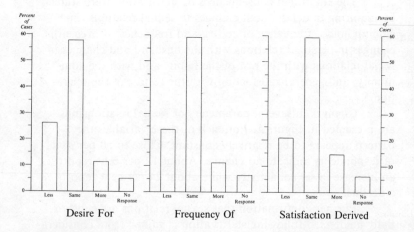

Fig. 1   Postoperative changes in desire for, frequency of, and satisfaction derived from sexual intercourse.

TABLE 8.   Changes in Personal Relations with the Husband, Rest of the Family, and Community.

	With Husband		With Rest of Family and Community	
	No.	%	No.	%
Better	56	10.8	0	0.0
Same	364	70.1	508	97.9
Worse	73	14.1	11	2.1
Not stated	26	5.0	0	0.0
Total	519	100.0	519	100.0

In respect to the patient-husband relationship it is not surprising to find that the changes reported are quite similar to those already cited in connection with sexual relations. There would appear little doubt that the operation had no significant effect in the patient's relationships with the rest of the family and with the community in general. This is probably caused by the general acceptance of sterilization in Puerto Rico as a routine surgical procedure.

Two further attempts were made to probe the extent and direction of psychological effects of sterilization. The patient was asked to describe her state of happiness after the operation as contrasted with before and then was requested to indicate whether or not she was satisfied with the operation. The results of these inquiries are shown in Table 9.

TABLE 9.   Changes in Relation to General Happiness after Operation.

	No.	%
Happier	360	69.4
As happy	116	22.3
Less happy	43	8.3
Total	519	100.0

TABLE 10.   Satisfaction with Results of Operation.

			No.	%
Satisfied			489	94.2
Not satisfied			28	5.3
Poorer health	7	1.3%		
Want more children	7	1.3%		
Problems in marriage	7	1.3%		
Knows of temporary				
contraception now	3	0.6%		
Religious beliefs	2	0.4%		
Home is wrecked	2	0.4%		
Not stated			2	0.4
Total			519	99.9

It is worth noting that nearly 70 per cent of the women who underwent sterilization claim to be happier than they were before, 22 per cent are as happy, and only slightly over 8 per cent are less happy in spite of the fact that most of the preceding tables show a somewhat reduced improvement in the particular relationship studied. In our opinion, the marked increase in happiness is the result of the freedom from fear of unwanted pregnancies.

In respect to Table 10, we would call attention to the high percentage of women who express satisfaction with the operation. This would appear to result largely from the judicious selection of candidates and the rejection of emotionally unstable, immature individuals acting on the spur of the moment.

In connection with the criteria for obtaining help from the Family Planning Association toward sterilization, the minimum age standards will undoubtedly seem very low in more conservative communities, but one must bear in mind that in Puerto Rico, as in most tropical countries, many young girls start reproducing around 15 or 16 and it is not uncommon to find 20-year-olds with 4 or 5 children. Under these circumstances, multiparity is considered more important than chronologic age as a criterion for sterilization.

FAILURE RATE

Although generally considered the safest contraceptive method, surgical sterilization is not 100 per cent effective. The percentage of failures varies with the surgical technique, other things being equal. In our series, different surgeons in different hospitals, with the use of different techniques, have all contributed in different proportions to the total sample. There were a total of 5 failures in 519 operations (less than 1 per cent as revealed by subsequent pregnancies), which in our opinion is a tolerable rate of failure.

COMMENT

Given a relatively young mother, an attained family size of 3 or more living children, limited economic resources, and a desire by both marital members to limit the size of their family to the achieved size, permanent control of fertility would appear to be a rational plan. Sterilization of the woman or man provides a procedure to gain such control.

The position of surgical sterilization in contraception control varies from one place to another. There appears to be a growing number of communities that accept sterilization as a proper procedure under defined circumstances which not infrequently include economic deprivation and multiparity.

In Puerto Rico we have been afforded an opportunity to study on a retrospective basis the medical and psychological sequelae of a large experience of the sterilization of women undertaken chiefly because of economic difficulties. It is probable that this is among the first such experiences reported, since most of the previous studies were primarily concerned with operations performed because of medical reasons.

The cases of sterilization in women studied were a sample of 519 patients, or 15.3 per cent, of 3,390 women sterilized under the auspices of the Family Planning Association of Puerto Rico from 1956 through 1961. The median age of the women was 30.1 years at time of operation, while the median number of living children was 3.7.

An examination of the medical records for the 3,390 cases of sterilization of women provides no evidence of loss of

life associated with the operation. A careful survey of records
of several private and government hospitals covering some
6,633 additional sterilizations of women failed to uncover a
single death. These findings are at variance with results reported by previous investigators. We are of the belief, however,
that when women are sterilized for other than medical complications of pregnancy and delivery, i.e., are essentially well, the
risk of death associated with interval tubal ligation may not
exceed 1 per 10,000, a most favorable outcome when contrasted
with the risk of death associated with ordinary childbirth,
which is approximately 5 to 10 per 10,000.

No immediate postoperative complications were reported
by 479 women, 92 per cent of the interviewed sample of
519. Wound infection was reported in 4 per cent of the cases.
Late sequelae of a physical nature proved difficult to assess. It
is of interest to note, however, that 42 per cent of the patients
reported an improvement in health following sterilization, 43
per cent reported no change, and 15 per cent reported a decline.

A detailed inquiry into the psychological consequences
of sterilization leads to the following three conclusions: sexual
relations are substantially not affected by sterilization; general
relationships between patient and husband and between patient
and community undergo changes which are not remarkably
different than those which might occur in the absence of sterilization; and the state of happiness of a group of sterilized
patients is significantly improved as a result of the operation.

Not infrequently considerable reservation about the
desirability of tubal ligation because of probable medical and
psychological sequelae can be noted in the literature (11).

We find no convincing evidence to support this attitude
when the patient population under consideration consists of
mothers who have attained a family size of three or more living
children, desire to limit their family to this number, and share
with their husband the desire to seek a permanent solution to
the problem of fertility control.

When contrasted with the alternative of 10 or more years
of contraception by constant use of hormone agents or mechan-

ical devices, sterilization, in view of our findings, hardly appears to be a procedure of extraordinary physical or psychological risk nor is its employment lacking in simple and clear logic.

SUMMARY

1. The results of a survey of medical and psychological sequelae among a sample of Puerto Rican women, sterilized from 1956 through 1961, has been presented.

2. At the time of sterilization the 519 women included in the study had a median age of 30.1 years, a median number of living children of 3.7, and were predominantly Catholic in religion.

3. The series here reported was concerned primarily with sterilizations performed for economic reasons.

4. No immediate postoperative physical complications were found in 92 per cent of the women studied. For those reporting complications 4 per cent involved cases of wound infection, 1 per cent were concerned with hemorrhage, and 3 per cent were ascribed to minor complications.

5. Psychological findings reported indicate that sexual relations are substantially not affected by sterilization, while the sterilized patients experience a marked improvement in their expressed level of happiness.

The authors wish to acknowledge the invaluable help of Mrs. Celestina Zalduondo and Mr. Luis A. Pérez de Jesús, Executive Director and Business Manager of the Family Planning Association of Puerto Rico, respectively, in the preparation of the questionnaire, the selection of interviewers, and the general conduct of the investigations.

REFERENCES

1. Shajaa, K.: Acta obst. gynec. scandinav. 12: 114, 1932.
2. Laws of Virginia: Chapter 451, 1962, Article No. 32, Sections 423-427.
3. Tietze, C., and Neuman, L.: Surgical Sterilization of Men and Women, New York, 1962, National Committee on Maternal Health, Publication No. 11.
4. Prystowsky, H., and Eastman, N. J.: J. A. M. A. 158: 463, 1955.
5. August, R. V.: Obst. & Gynec. 5: 715, 1955.
6. Flowers, C. E., Donnelly, J. F., and Burwell, J. C.: North Carolina M. J. 20: 489, 1959.

7. Berthelson, H. G.: Danish M. Bull. 4: 107, 1957.
8. Naville, A.: Praxis 41: 1020, 1952.
9. De, Nagandraneth: J. Indian M. A. 36: 95, 1961.
10. Barnes, A. C., and Zuspan, F. P.: Am. J. Obst. & Gynec. 75: 65, 1958.
11. Swartz, D. P., et al.: Fertil. & Steril. 14: 320, 1963.

4   VOLUNTARY STERILIZATION — A WORLD VIEW

by Harriet B. Presser

Other than sterility, what changes occur to persons who undergo the operation? Different studies ask this question in different ways, but three areas of concern provide a basis for making comparisons. These areas are: general satisfaction with the operation, change in sexual desire or activity, and change in general health. They will be considered separately for male and female sterilization because it is of interest to see whether a differential effect is reported by sex. It should be noted that most of the replies are retrospective evaluations made by respondents, and the time period since sterilization varies by study. Without a control group of nonsterilized persons, it is difficult to assess the extent to which some changes would have occurred over time without sterilization even though respondents attribute such changes to the operation.

GENERAL SATISFACTION

A large majority of men in the studies reported in Table 1 expressed satisfaction with vasectomy; the range is from 68 to 100 per cent. There is considerable variation within country by study, but it appears that males in the United States are more satisfied with vasectomy than males in India or Pakistan. Perhaps this has to do with the fact that the infant and child mortality rate in the United States is not so high as in Pakistan and India. As noted earlier, a major reason for seeking a reversal operation is the death of children — which is less likely to occur in the United States. Another important reason for seeking a reversal operation is remarriage. As adult mortality is also not so high in the United States as in Pakistan

TABLE 1. Per Cent of Sterilized Males Reporting Satisfaction with Vasectomy, for Three Specified Countries (Limited to studies published in 1960 or later)

Country and Subnational Area	Year of Publication	Author	Number Reporting on Satisfaction	Per Cent Satisfied
India				
Gujarat	1963	Poffenberger and Sheth	61	87
Jammu and Kashmir	1969	Sawhney and Langoo	175	68
Maharashtra	1963[a]	Dandekar	1,191	92
Pakistan				
East	1969	Quddus et al.	135	87
West	1968	Ilahi	60	98
United States				
California	1963	Poffenberger and Poffenberger	29	100
California	1964	Ziegler et al.	44	100
Minnesota	1965	Truesdale	137	98
Washington	1964	Johnson	83	80
Ten urban areas [b]	1967	Ferber et al.	73	99

[a] Including small proportions in some studies indicating indifference or no opinion.
[b] Majority in sample from New York City.

Source: Derived from data given in abbreviated citations shown above. For full citation, see References.

and India, we may infer that proportionately more vasectomized males in Pakistan and India are likely to regret sterilization because of the death of the wife than are likely to in the United States. On the other hand, marital instability is higher in the United States than in the other two countries. Accordingly, regret because of remarriage and the desire for additional children may be about equally likely in the three countries.

Table 2 reveals that the large majority of sterilized women, like sterilized men, are satisfied with the operation. The per cent satisfied with tubal sterilization in these studies ranges from 78 to 99. It may be noted that the developing countries rank among the highest in satisfaction with tubal sterilization, despite their high infant mortality rates. The lower rates of satisfaction for some of the developed countries may have to do, at least in part, with psychological selectivity. Many women

TABLE 2.   Per Cent of Sterilized Females Reporting Satisfaction with Tubal Sterilization, for Eight Specified Countries (Limited to studies published in 1960 or later)

Country and Subnational Area	Year of Publication	Author	Number Reporting on Satisfaction	Per Cent Satisfied [a]
Ceylon	1963	Chinnatamby	412	98
England	1968	Thompson	186	87
Finland	1964	Rauramo and Paavola	542	87
Hong Kong [b]	1967	Lu and Chun	1,055	99
India				
Andhra Pradesh	1968	H. K. Rao et. al.	160	96
Maharashtra	1964	Coyaji	839	97
Maharashtra	1966	Ghatikar and Bhoopatkar	520	97
Puerto Rico [b]	1964	Paniagua et al.	519	94
Sweden	1961	Ekblad	225	78
	1965	Kaij and Malmquist	179	79
United States				
Iowa	1964	Norris	88	91[c]
Oregon	1964	Adams [d]	107[e]	97
Oregon	1964	Adams [d]	65[f]	99

[a] Including small proportions in some studies indicating indifference or no opinion.
[b] Nonsovereign territory.
[c] Including 17 per cent who indicated "occasional regret" but nevertheless were "glad" the operation had been done.
[d] Study limited to those sterilized for socioeconomic reasons only.

[e] First follow-up, one to three years after sterilization.
[f] Second follow-up, four to seven years after sterilization.
Source: Derived from data given in abbreviated citations shown above. For full citation, see References.

in the Swedish studies, for example, were sterilized for psychiatric reasons (Ekblad, 1961; Kaij and Malmquist, 1965). Although such women practiced sterilization voluntarily as a means of birth control, we would expect them to be less satisfied with the operation than women without psychiatric problems.

CHANGE IN SEXUAL DESIRE OR ACTIVITY

Biologically, there does not appear to be any reason why sterilization should affect sexual desire or activity. Psychologically, however, there are several reasons. We would expect sexual desire and activity to increase after sterilization if the fear of pregnancy had previously been a deterrent to such activity. On the other hand, if there is not a full understanding of the operation, subsequent sexual behavior may be restricted. Fears of impotence and negative reactions to barrenness may reduce one's interest in sex; these may be particularly true of persons sterilized for psychiatric reasons. It should also be kept in mind that persons age during the years following sterilization and, insofar as aging is associated with a decrease in sexual desire and activity, a decrease following sterilization cannot be attributed solely to the operation. Other personal factors may also be responsible for any change. Again, what is needed for comparison but missing in these studies is a control group of nonsterilized persons.

Table 3 reveals that, in most studies, a majority of men report no change in sexual desire or activity following vasectomy; there is, however, substantial variation in the percentage by study both within and between countries and states. The range reporting no change is from 35 to 83 per cent. For those reporting a change, there does not appear to be an overall consistent pattern in the direction of the change. Some studies show large increases in sexual behavior or desire after vasectomy (e.g., in Poffenberger and Poffenberger, 1963, an increase of 48 per cent), while others show large decreases (e.g., in Dandekar, 1963b, a decrease of 54 per cent). Even within subsamples of a single study of Korean men (Lee, 1966), there is some difference in the sexual effects of vasectomy; proportionately fewer private patients indicated a decrease in sexual desire or activity than did subsidized patients.

Studies of sterilized women also show considerable variation by country in changes in sexual desire or activity after sterilization (Table 4); there are too few studies to consider within-country differences. Substantial increases in sexual desire or activity after tubal sterilization were reported in the Swedish (Kaij and Malmquist, 1965) and English (Thompson, 1968) studies: 29 and 44 per cent, respectively. Substantial decreases ranging from 22 per cent to 36 per cent may be noted

TABLE 3. Per Cent Distribution of Sterilized Males, by Reported Changes in Sexual Desire or Activity, for Four Specified Countries (Limited to studies published in 1960 or later)

Country and Subnational Area	Year of Publication	Author	Per cent distribution by reported changes in sexual desire or activity				Total	
			No Change	Increase	Decrease	No Response	Per Cent	Number
India								
Delhi	1964	Bhatnagar	69	19	12	0	100	330
Delhi	1968	Sandhu and Bhardwaj	57	16	23	4	100	146
Gujarat	1963	Poffenberger and Sheth	59	15	10	16	100	61
Madhya Pradesh	1968	Halder	60	12	23	5	100	250
Maharashtra	1961[b]	Phadke	80	12	8	0	100	655
Maharashtra	1963[b]	Dandekar	35	11	54	0	100	1,191
Mysore and Tamil Nadu[a]	1968[b]	H. K. Rao	83	4	7	6	100	247
Uttar Pradesh	1961	Banerji	54	39	7	0	100	202
Korea (Republic of)								
	1966	Lee	81	14	5	0	100	320[b]
	1966	Lee	71	14	11	4	100	3,413[c]
Pakistan								
East	1969	Islam	65	5	30	0	100	113
East	1969	Mannan	44	15	27	14	100	100
West	1968	Ilahi	82	15	3	0	100	60
West	1969	Quddus et al.	59	9	29	3	100	135
United States								
California	1963	Landis and Poffenberger	60	38	2	0	100	330
California	1963	Poffenberger and Poffenberger	62	38	0	0	100	29
California	1964	Ziegler et al.	56	40	4	0	100	44
Minnesota	1965	Truesdale	73	24	3	0	100	137
Washington	1964	Johnson	0	15	13	72	100	83

[a] Formerly Madras.
[b] Private patients.
[c] Subsidized patients.

Source: Derived from data given in abbreviated citations shown above. For full citation, see References.

TABLE 4.   Per Cent Distribution of Sterilized Females, by Reported Changes in Sexual Desire or Activity, for Six Specified Countries
(Limited to studies published in 1960 or later)

Country and Subnational Area	Year of Publication	Author	Per cent distribution by reported changes in sexual desire or activity					Total Number
			No Change	Increase	Decrease	No Response	Per Cent	
Ceylon	1963	Chinnatamby	60	4	36	0	100	412
England	1968	Thompson	40	44	11	5	100	186
Finland	1964	Rauramo and Paavola	63	8	22	7	100	542
India								
Andhra Pradesh	1968	H. K. Rao et al.	0	8	16	76[a]	100	160
West Bengal	1966	Dawn	0	0	11	89[b]	100	42
Puerto Rico [c]	1964	Paniagua et al.	60	12	24	4	100	519
Sweden	1965	Kaij and Malmquist	60	29	11	0	100	178

[a] Study gives only the number who reported an increase or decrease in sexual desire or activity; it is not possible to distinguish nonresponse from no change.

[b] Study gives only the number who reported a decrease in sexual desire or activity.

[c] Nonsovereign territory.

Source: Derived from data given in abbreviated citations shown above. For full citation, see References.

for studies of sterilized women in Finland (Rauramo and Paavola, 1964), Puerto Rico (Paniagua et al., 1964), and Ceylon (Chinnatamby, 1963). The two Indian studies do not report their data in a way that is comparable to the other studies, making it difficult to rank them accordingly.

These data suggest that a relatively high prevalence of male sterilization (India) or female sterilization (Puerto Rico) is not correlated with an especially high percentage reporting no change or an increase in sexual desire or activity after sterilization. Studies in these countries do not show the highest percentages satisfied with sterilization either (see Tables 1 and 2). The data also do not lead to any conclusions about differences in the sexual effects of male and female sterilization.

Part Seven ♀♂

Vasectomy: Reversibility and Frozen Semen Banks

1 THE REVERSIBILITY OF MALE STERILIZATION

by Joseph E. Davis, M.D.

If male sterilization were truly a reversible operation, we would more properly speak of it as a male contraceptive procedure performed by surgical means. Bilateral vasectomy simply interrupts the passage of sperm through the male tube called the vas deferens. However, the significance of the interruption of the duct on each side is of greater complexity than was formerly thought. As a result, numerous researchers are working towards the development of a new procedure — a simple technique for reversing the occlusion. When this is achieved, we will have a contraceptive type of operation, and the term "sterilization" will disappear from use. Whatever the device or technique, it will easily be reversed by a second operation, or conceivably by the use of an external magnet that will allow the patient to "turn off" and "turn on." The operation then would hopefully be no more difficult than the insertion of an intra-uterine device (IUD) into the female.

It is clear that sterilization will not be an important factor in the control of population until such techniques make the operation reversible. The number seeking temporary surgical sterilization will probably be larger than those seeking an irreversible operation today.

The criterion for true reversibility would be an operation simply performed — the insertion of some device into each tube which would cause little reaction locally or generally in the body, and could easily be removed at a second operation with little untoward effect on the patient. Such an operation would impede sperm, and on removal would allow sperm to go through the tube easily. In addition, there would be no damage to the fertilizing capacity of the sperm.

The growing reports of reversibility so far have considered the passage of sperm through the operated area as indicative of success. On this basis, success rates range from 50 to 90 per cent. However, fertility rates are not as high. In the latest series reported at the American Fertility Society (New Orleans, La., 1971) a potency rate of only 25 per cent was reported in over 400 men who underwent reestablishment of the continuity of the duct system. Until an operation is devised that will give an 80 to 90 per cent fertility rate afterwards, we will fall short of true reversibility.

THE ANATOMY AND PHYSIOLOGY OF THE MALE DUCT SYSTEM AND EFFECTS OF VAS SURGERY

Until recently it was thought that the male tube which conducts sperm was simply a conduit for millions of sperm produced each day. But new research shows that the vas deferens is constantly in motion due to the nerve supply, which causes peristaltic activity. Wave-like motions of the vas deferens are under the control of the nervous system of the body. During ejaculation, sperm are forced up this tube from the testicles and epididymis, probably under great pressure. One only has to examine the human vas to see that it has a thick, complex muscular wall which undoubtedly forces large amounts of sperm up the canal during ejaculation.

When the vas deferens is cut during vasectomy, most surgeons remove a significant piece, that is, from 1 to 5 cm. (the vas deferens is 18 cm. in length). It is evident that some damage must be done to the nervous system and to the ability of this structure to propel sperm. No studies are available that indicate the effects of vasectomy upon the function of the vas, but there are studies which indicate that some loss of normal function probably occurs during the operation.

After sperm are blocked by vasectomy from passing up the tube, sperm nevertheless continue to be produced by the testicle and pass through the epididymis where many are absorbed into the general body system. Yet some sperm probably attempt to move up the blind end of the cut and tied tube. If the tying is not secure, or if there is destruction of the area around the suture, sperm may leak and cause a tissue reaction (or sperm granuloma). This may set up a reaction of the body producing antibodies, and cause an immune reaction with a foreign body now present — that is, the sperm outside the normal duct system. If this occurs, sperm antibodies may be found circulating in the blood stream. It is not known whether these antibodies have any significant or ill effects upon the body, but it is thought that many men may become infertile as a result.

Thus, vasectomy may cause an immune phenomenon — the antibodies' response to the body, which may render the male infertile at a later date even though successful reestablishment of continuity of the vas deferens has been achieved.

Less understood are the effects of closing off this tube on the structure of the sperm subsequently produced or their fertilizing capacity. The response might be the same if temporary devices were used. Therefore, research now in progress must determine the effect of occlusion, whether permanent or temporary. Until the effects of occlusion and effects upon the testicles are known, we will still not have the answer to reversibility in spite of the most sophisticated temporary devices which may be developed.

TECHNIQUES FOR REVERSIBILITY

Surgical reanastomosis of the vasectomized individual has been the standard approach to reversibility in the past. The surgeon must reoperate, cut away the scar tissue at the site of the previous operation, and determine if there is complete patency of the tube from below and above. Usually sperm fluid will pass up the lower end upon pressure on the epididymis. Sperm are then searched for under a microscope, and if they are found, the surgeon proceeds to sew together the two ends of the vas deferens, usually using an operating microscope for careful approximation of the two ends.

Since there is the chance of scarring in the area, most surgeons use a splint across the new opening for a period between 8 to 10 days. The splint, made of either metal or nylon, is removed through a blind end below the operative site. Other surgeons prefer to leave no splint in the area of joining.

External clips. The tantalum clip has been used recently for external occlusion. This has been studied in dogs, but the results were only fair. With one clip, sperm got through the site of the occlusion. With two clips, there was such damage to the wall of the vas deferens that upon removal of the clips, the sperm would not pass through. Newer clips are being developed which do not cause as much damage, and this type of external occlusion may prove a simple way of providing reversibility after a second operation to remove the clips.

Intravasal materials. Numerous materials have been suggested to occlude sperm: various plastics, silicone, polyethylene, Barium Ferrite, stainless steel, and tantalum. These materials have not been thoroughly tested. With plastics there is a problem of migration from the area of occlusion; with other substances there is a question of tissue reaction and effect upon the sperm. These are still experimental and a large amount of work must be done on animals before application to human beings.

Intravasal valves. Microvalves have been developed which may prove the answer to the problem of reversibility. Microvalves may be set in the "on" and "off" position. They usually have stems that can be turned with a fine needle. They may be inserted into a small opening usually made in a longitudinal direction in the vas deferens. The stem generally protrudes from the vas, and thus fixes the vas in a particular area, preventing migration. The valve is sewn into place. If the male desires the valve turned into an "on" position, a second operation is required.

After extensive valve tests in our laboratory with guinea pigs (an animal readily studied in terms of determining the point of disappearance and reappearance of sperm following valve turnings), the tests were most rewarding in achieving successful reversibility. This work is now being applied to human volunteers. Hopefully, within three to five years the microvalve will be a valuable contribution to the heretofore insoluble problem of reversibility.

Intravasal threads or sutures. Several investigators, particularly Dr. Hee Yong Lee of Korea, have had extensive experience with threads passed through one wall of the vas, out another wall, and tied around the vas. The intravasal portion of the thread serves as the occlusion. The reversal operation simply removes the thread. Results in these cases have been excellent. Reversal, measured by the return of sperm in the ejaculate following removal, has achieved about 90 per cent success. Return of sperm usually occurred around one month after reversal. Yet the patency rate in men who were reversed is no higher than with standard reversal operations already described.

RESULTS
Analyzing the results of standard surgical reversal, one investigator who has done numerous reanastomosis operations concludes, "Although the great majority of patients show live active sperm in their ejaculate immediately following the operation, and for as long as two years after the operation, late scar formation will occasionally block the vas after two or more years of patency."

This is due to an anatomical fact. While the overall diameter of the vas deferens is quite large (approximately the size of a wax pencil), the lumen through which the sperm flows is very tiny, smaller than the smallest milliner's needle. The lumen may thus be occluded by a tiny scar. Because of the possibility of occlusion a few years after reversal, it has been suggested that attempts at pregnancy be made soon after the reversal operation prior to the redevelopment of scarring. Fortunately, men with vasectomies often have two or three children and proven fertility. Even if only a small number of sperm get through the operative site, their sperm is apparently of a high degree of fertility, increasing the chances of a successful outcome.

In the hands of the experienced surgeon, the success rate of getting sperm through the operative site has been about 60 to 80 per cent. The pregnancy rate, however, is only about 20 to 30 per cent.

We still do not know whether newer techniques will improve the success rate of reversibility. The value of these techniques depends upon how minimally they affect the anatomy of the tube, how well they prevent sperm from escaping from the area of surgery, and how little the device damages motility and normal functioning of the vas deferens.

SPERM BANKS: THE FIRST STEP TO REVERSIBILITY

The freezing and storage of semen from patients before vasectomy is a practical procedure that can now be used to overcome the drawbacks of permanent sterilization. This is an important breakthrough, preserving the fertility potential of men who formerly had to undergo irreversible operations. The establishment of semen banks will remove the onus of fertility loss. Even though only a small number of vasectomy applicants seek to store their semen, the knowledge that the bank has removed this major drawback of fertility loss should act as an incentive to the increased choice of vasectomy. The use of the semen bank may be presented to the potential vasectomy patient as a form of "fertility insurance." It should provide a significant impetus that will greatly increase the appeal of vasectomy or other types of reversible male sterilization. Now men can have the use-effectiveness of vasectomy plus the retention of their fertility potential.

The ability to freeze human semen and subsequently defrost it and still preserve the normal fertilizing capacity of the sperm has been available since 1960. Over 300 children have been born by artificial insemination of the female, using previously frozen semen which has been stored for periods of one to ten years. No abnormalities in fetal growth or in the development of the children have been reported. New techniques have made sperm freezing commercially valuable.

We have no accurate statistics on how many men will request reversal by any type of surgical procedure — no more than one to five out of 1,000 according to present studies. Perhaps the rate will increase with advances in reversible operations, and increase even further with the effect of sperm banks. Yet the availability of surgical reversibility and semen banks will no doubt sharply intensify the total demand for vasectomy.

If reversibility is truly available, the word "sterilization" can then be eliminated from the vocabulary of the family planner and population control expert.

2   THE USE OF FROZEN SEMEN BANKS TO PRESERVE THE FERTILITY OF VASECTOMIZED MEN

by Matthew Freund, Ph.D.

A frozen semen bank, which contains the viable sperm of men who have used vasectomy for contraception, represents a true method for reversible vasectomy in terms of perpetuating the fertility of the vasectomized man. Inasmuch as the man retains his potency and his potential fertility (in terms of frozen sperm) after vasectomy, this technique will remove the onus of loss of fertility from the vasectomy operation. Frozen semen banks will indefinitely preserve the fertility of men undergoing vasectomy. The provision of frozen semen banks should act as an incentive for the increased use of vasectomy for contraception since it removes the major drawback of permanent loss of fertility. From an acceptance-of-contraception point of view, the use of frozen semen banks as a backup for vasectomy should provide a dramatic and popular impetus that will vastly increase the appeal of vasectomy as a method of contraception. Indeed, with frozen semen as a form of fertility insurance, the concept of vasectomy as a "sterilization" operation should give way to that of vasectomy as a "contraceptive" operation.

While it is evident how semen banks may be set up and used in developed countries such as the United States, their potential use in developing countries may be even more important from the point of view of world population control and must be seriously considered.

The freezing and storage of semen from vasectomy patients is a practical procedure that can be used at this time to overcome the drawbacks of vasectomy. I must be recognized that workers in the field of family planning may balk at the idea of the administrative difficulties and financial investment involved in setting up frozen semen banks in developing countries. However, the relative safety, use-effectiveness, and cost-effectiveness of vasectomy with a frozen semen bank backup must be carefully compared with that of the conventional, presently available, contraceptives. It is my belief that the single application of vasectomy plus frozen semen (for that percentage of men who want this fertility insurance) will prove more practical and cheaper, in the long run, than the creation and maintenance of a medical and social infrastructure to deliver repeated applications of conventional contraception. Realistic costing of relative use-effectiveness and cost-effectiveness that includes the critical elements of safety and efficacy must be applied to determine the relative value of vasectomy plus frozen semen banks.

Even though only a relatively small number of the men who have had a vasectomy for contraception may seek to use the fertility potential in their stored semen, the knowledge that the semen bank has removed the major drawback of permanent loss of fertility from the vasectomy procedure should act as an incentive for the increased choice of vasectomy for contraception. The use of a frozen semen bank will be presented to the potential vasectomy patient as a form of "fertility insurance."

In this laboratory, human sperm have been successfully diluted, frozen, and stored at -196°C. (under the surface of liquid nitrogen) for periods of up to four years without loss of motility. We plan to correlate and coordinate our studies on vasectomy with concurrent studies on frozen human semen. We will create a frozen semen bank and will measure the fertility of frozen diluted human semen over long periods of time — decades. We propose to lead the way to frozen semen banks that will preserve the fertility potential of men undergoing vasectomy for contraception and, at the same time, do a whole spectrum of quantitative studies in human reproductive physiology. It is planned to use the frozen semen for artificial insemination in carefully controlled experimental designs so as to provide a semen bank that contains sperm of known genetic and fertility quality for the most benefit in donor insemination and so as to yield maximum information on the mechanisms of sperm migration and viability in the female reproductive tract and on the physiology of fertilization in man (see Note I, below).

The improvements and refinements in the methods for dilution, cooling, freezing, storage, and defrosting led to increasing recoveries of motile sperm until we were able to report a standardized technique for essentially complete recovery of motility upon defrosting. Human semen may be successfully and routinely diluted, frozen, and stored provided that a sequence of critical steps is carefully followed. To date, methods of freezing and storage developed in this laboratory have permitted us to preserve the motility of human sperm for 48 months, which was the duration of that particular research study. It is anticipated that the motility and fertility of frozen diluted human semen stored at -196° C. under the surface of liquid nitrogen can be preserved indefinitely. Bull semen has been preserved for more than 10 years without loss of fertility and the same should be true of human semen. Indeed, it is possible to predict on theoretical grounds that human sperm could be preserved indefinitely at -196° C. — perhaps "forever."

From our data, which indicate no decline in motility over a four-year storage period, it is possible to predict theoretically that human sperm could be preserved indefinitely at -196° C. However, this must be shown directly and empirically by storage experiments lasting at least 10 years with examination for motility and fertility at yearly intervals. The successful storage of diluted human semen with retention of motility and fertility for a period of 10 years should allow us to directly predict that human sperm could be preserved indefinitely in ampules under the surface of liquid nitrogen (see Note II, below).

A basic premise in our work is that *diluted* human semen must be used in order to make possible critical and quantitative studies. The important scientific achievements resulting from the use of frozen bull semen are based on the fact that methods have been developed to dilute bull semen without marked loss of viability or fertility so that, after the freezing and storage of the diluted semen, it is possible to inseminate a large number of cows with the sperm from a single ejaculate. The preparation of many ampules of frozen diluted semen from a single ejaculate makes it practical to replicate so that 1) duplicate ampules may be prepared and examined at intervals, 2) treatment effects may be quantitatively measured, and 3) the variance among ampules treated alike may be used as an error term to test for the significance of treatment differences.

Recently, Bunge summed up his experience with frozen semen ("9 drops of liquefied semen and 1 drop of glycerol"), as follows: "We have used frozen spermatozoa many times and have derived over 100 children from these inseminations. In none has there been a disease, disorder, or anomaly attributable to the freezing. I have not reported this series because I deem it of the utmost significance that at least one of these children should reproduce and the progeny be critically examined. However, at this time I shall show you a photograph of one of our older children born of frozen semen. He is a 16-year-old boy, 6 feet tall, in excellent health, and an A student."

The important report by Iizuka, Sawada, Nishina, and Ohi is apparently the first quantitative and statistical report of a follow-up study on children born as a result of artificial insemination with frozen semen. They examined 46 children and found that their physical and mental development was normal in every respect and comparable to a control group of children. At the June 1971, convention of The American Medical Association, Dr. Edward T. Tyler described a series of 68 children born as a result of insemination with frozen semen. These workers have clearly shown that undiluted frozen human semen can be successfully used for artificial insemination and that the pregnancies and the children are normal in every respect.

Thus these studies with raw semen are basic to the field, although it is difficult to see how they can be applied to the development of practical semen banks on a large scale or to research studies on the physiology of reproduction in man. Studies based on frozen raw (undiluted) human semen must remain qualitative or, at best, semiquantitative since there is not enough volume in a single ejaculate (1-4 ml.) to permit treatment replication or the calculation of an error term. Frozen raw human semen is essentially a fascinating scientific curiosity which can be used to produce a limited number of conceptions. The use of *frozen diluted* human semen is a prerequisite for large-scale, practical, efficient frozen semen banks in man (just as it was in dairy cattle). The use of frozen diluted human semen will lead to controlled and replicated scientific investigations and to practical studies of semen fertility in artificial insemination.

The good fertility of frozen human semen has been clearly demonstrated by the birth of almost 500 children throughout the world. However, most of this work has been done by individual physicians and, therefore, has had little or no impact on the progress of family planning. It seems evident that there is now a need for a scale up of the freezing and storage of human semen so that its use as a practical backup for vasectomies may aid in the program to educate men to the simplicity and effectiveness of vasectomy as a method of family planning. To this end, a new national corporation based in New York City, Idant Corporation, has been formed to fill this need and to provide semen banks for the long-term storage of semen from vasectomy patients. It is believed that this national service to preserve the fertility of vasectomized men, based in many cities in this country and eventually around the world, will make a significant contribution to family planning and to the solution of the population explosion.*

*Idant's approximate price for the tests and storage of sperm for six months is $80; then a charge of about $40 for three years, $18 for one year, if the man decides to continue storage.

SUMMARY

The long-term storage of semen from vasectomy patients represents a true method for reversible vasectomy in terms of perpetuating the fertility of the vasectomized man. This option will be offered to each of the patients who volunteers for vasectomy and the results of this study should point the way towards the mass application of frozen semen banks as an incentive for the increased use of vasectomy, since it removes the major drawback of loss of fertility. The use of a frozen semen bank will be presented to the potential vasectomy patient as a form of "fertility insurance." It should provide a dramatic and popular argument for vasectomy that will vastly increase the appeal of vasectomy as a method of contraception.

Notes

I. The effects of and interactions among the many factors affecting the dilution, cooling, freezing, storage, and defrosting of human semen were investigated and reported. The factors studied included buffers and diluters, dilution rate, rate of cooling (+20° C. to +5° C.), "cold shock," cryoprotective effects of glycerol and egg yolk, rate of cooling (+5° C. to -70° C.), method of cooling (dry ice, liquid nitrogen vapor, isopropyl alcohol), storage temperature (-79° C., -85° C., -196° C.), length of storage, and rate of defrosting.

A tissue-culture medium, such as Norman-Johnson solution, must be used for dilution (1:5, 1:10, and 1:20) since human spermatozoa rapidly lose their motility upon dilution with the conventional phosphate or citrate diluents used with bull semen. Egg yolk (10%) and glycerol (7%) are essential to prevent respectively cold shock and freezing damage. Slow cooling from +20° C. to +5° C. over a period of three hours is required to prevent cold shock and subsequent loss of motility. The diluted semen must be frozen in 1-ml quantities in ampules at an average and constant rate of -1° C./min from +5° to -70° C. The frozen semen must be stored at -196° C., since it shows a steady loss of motility with time when stored at -79° C. to -85° C. The semen must be slowly defrosted to +20° C. in air over a period of 15 minutes, since defrosting over a 3- to 5-minute period in water bath at +5° C., +25° C., or +37° C. causes a severe drop in per cent motility. These steps constitute a standardized and repeatable technique for the dilution, freezing, and long-term storage (up to 48 months) of human spermatozoa with essentially complete recovery of motility upon defrosting.

II. The fertility of frozen semen used in artificial insemination must be compared against a control; in this case, the fertility of fresh semen used in artificial insemination. Sawada and Behrman attempted to do this by inseminating with frozen semen for several cycles and then, in those women who failed to conceive, inseminating with fresh semen for several cycles. The drawbacks to this procedure are evident because the different semen specimen used in each case and the decrease in average fertility of the group of selected women who failed to get pregnant as the study progressed, served to confound the direct comparison between frozen and fresh semen.

We propose to make this comparison in three ways. In the first way, this would be done by splitting each specimen and using half the doses of insemination as fresh semen and the other half for freezing and storage and then for insemination as frozen semen; conceivably, this study could be done as a "double blind." In the second way, this would be done by using alternate specimens of a donor for insemination with fresh semen or for insemination with frozen semen; again, this study could be done as a "double blind" by putting the fresh semen into ampules before delivering it to the physician. In the third way, the fertility of the frozen semen from a vasectomy patient would be compared to the fertility of the same donor before vasectomy. In some cases this comparison would be made on the same woman and in other cases on different women. Particular attention will be paid to the possibility of diluting and cooling human semen to +5°C. and then maintaining it for several days at +5°C. This has been done successfully in the bull and the diluted and cooled semen retains its motility and fertility for several days. If this is practical with human semen, it will give us a much more statistically meaningful number of inseminations with fresh semen as a control.

We have shown that frozen diluted human semen must be stored at -196°C., under the surface of liquid nitrogen, since it shows a steady loss of motility with time when stored at -79°C. or at -85°C. So far, we have kept 25 specimens under the surface of liquid nitrogen for 48 months without loss of motility.

Part Eight ⚥

Voluntary Sterilization: How to Find the Best Doctor, Clinic, or Hospital at the Most Reasonable Price

1 THE STRUCTURE OF A LARGE-SCALE VASECTOMY CLINIC

by Abel J. Leader, M.D.

No single factor has so stimulated the growth of voluntary sterilization as the out-patient vasectomy clinic. Since 1969, when the Association for Voluntary Sterilization made the initial grant for the Margaret Sanger Research Bureau clinic in New York, 175 similar clinics have sprung up across the country in 32 states. With new clinics opening regularly, vasectomy should be available to almost every man near his home city or town within a few years.

Because of its long established network of chapters and clinics, Planned Parenthood's recent support provides a significant boost to sterilization. Many Planned Parenthood clinics have now added vasectomy services. In this article, Dr. Abel J. Leader describes how Planned Parenthood of Houston, Texas, organized and runs its vasectomy program.

It may seem heretical to say so, but it cannot be seriously argued, nor is it frivolous to say, that in its potential impact on the sum total of human happiness and of the future of mankind, this simple operation of vasectomy is of enormous consequence.

It must be made readily available to all who seek it.

The principal stimulus leading to the development of the Vasectomy Clinic of Planned Parenthood of Houston was the unfair and unfavorable publicity given the steroid pill during the course of the Nelson Senate Committee hearings in early 1970. Couples who considered their families complete began to question the wisdom of continuing to use the pill, intrauterine devices, or other contraceptive measures whose failure rates were disquieting. Many inquiries were then received by the Affiliate in Houston regarding vasectomy. Mr. Norman Fleischman, then the Executive Director of the Center, turned to Dr. Jack Moore, at that time Chairman of the Medical Advisory Committee, for help.

As elsewhere, vasectomy had been done in doctors' offices for the purpose of effecting sterilization for many years, but in no great numbers. There were several reasons for this:

1. Almost all hospital by-laws prohibited sterilization for other than valid medical reasons. These usually required one or more consultations corroborating the medical necessity for the procedure. Social and economic considerations carried no weight.

2. For reasons of religious conscience, many physicians refused to perform vasectomy, when the primary purpose was to effect sterilization, either in the hospital or in their offices. Vasectomy incidental to prostatectomy, for the purpose of preventing postoperative epidiymitis was permitted.

3. Because of their antipathy on religious grounds to sterilization, many such physicians communicated to their inquiring patients a distorted and unfounded concern for possible adverse sexual, psychic, and physiologic consequences of vasectomy. Some patients were boldly told that the procedure was illegal and constituted mayhem; at the least, others were made to feel that they had asked for the male equivalent of a criminal abortion.

4. Many other urologists, even if willing to perform office vasectomy, found that the initial interview, in which the physician was expected to answer the many questions asked concerning the procedure by the patient and his spouse, was enormously time consuming, taking up more time than he could spare from

a busy day. Many of these people were "shoppers" and as many as a third of these people were "drop-outs," making negative decisions.

5. Physicians, even if willing to perform vasectomy in their offices, had widely varying sets of standards for eligibility for vasectomy, relating to the age of the patients, the number of children in the family, etc. In other words, they would "play God," and this added to the difficulty in referring patients for the procedure.

6. In an age of increasing malpractice litigation, the performance of vasectomy left many physicians who might otherwise have done the procedure in their offices wary of such consequences. This, despite the fact that vasectomy is associated with less such harassment than any other surgical procedure.

7. Many urologists in Houston, recognizing that the individual patient who appears in their offices has his Freudian complexes sticking out all over, are now convinced that the procedure is best done in a clinic atmosphere — on the basis that 10-20 patients gathered for a common purpose find mutual reassurance and the moral courage that might otherwise be lacking. Many of the referrals to the Vasectomy Clinic are made by these urologists, without regard to the economic status of the patient.

8. Finally, for many, the fee for an office vasectomy has been higher than many can afford to pay.

Dr. Jack Moore made an appearance, on invitation, before the Houston Urological Society, asking for the cooperation of all urologists in the matter of establishing a vasectomy referral service for the Planned Parenthood Center. By unanimous vote such cooperation was pledged, and a committee headed by Dr. Russell Scott, Chairman of the Department of Urology at Baylor, was appointed to act in this matter.

Originally intending only to develop a referral roster that might be used by the Center, it became apparent to the committee that a vasectomy service to care for low income groups should also be a part of the program. The referral roster was to be composed of the responses of the urologists to a questionnaire sent with the following covering letter:

Dear Doctor: A tremendous increase in the number of requests for, and information concerning vasectomy has prompted Planned Parenthood of Houston, with the cooperation of the Houston Urological Society, to set up a Vasectomy Clinic in the near future. This is intended to serve low income groups primarily.

It is expected that Planned Parenthood of Houston's Clinic will receive many inquiries from patients who would prefer to consult and can afford to pay a private physician for this service.

In anticipation of this, we are preparing a roster of physicians to whom such patients may be referred. This letter and questionnaire seeks an expression of your interest and of your views on the subject of vasectomy.

We should like to conserve your time, that of your staff, and of the staff of our Clinic by referring to you only those patients for whom you are willing to do this procedure as an out-patient. Your prompt reply will be appreciated.

The questionnaire sent to all members of the Houston Urological Society is shown here:

QUESTIONNAIRE ON VASECTOMY

1. Do you perform vasectomy upon request as an office procedure?   Yes __   No __ .

2. Because this question is almost always asked and because we wish to avoid wasting your time with "shoppers," what is your fee or range of fees for this procedure? $ ____ to $ ____ .

3. Do you wish your name placed on Planned Parenthood's roster of physicians to whom patients may be referred? Yes __   No __ .

4. Usually the patient is required to pay the fee for this procedure before or at the time the vasectomy is done. Is this your practice, also?   Yes __   No __ . Or may the pa-

tient make arrangements with your office to pay this fee at a later time: Yes ___   No ___ ; or in installments: Yes ___   No ___ .

5.   The earliest age at which you will perform vasectomy, the patient's wife concurring, and reservations you have as to family size, is as follows: (Please indicate by appropriate check-mark or by circling numbers).

Age Range	Won't Do at All	Will Do Without Reservation	Will Do but Only with at Least This Number of Children					
20-25	_____	_____	1	2	3	4	5	6
26-30	_____	_____	1	2	3	4	5	6
31-35	_____	_____	1	2	3	4	5	6
36-40	_____	_____	1	2	3	4	5	6
41-50	_____	_____	1	2	3	4	5	6

6.   Would you perform vasectomy on a single man, or a married man with no children (the latter's wife concurring) with a history of congenital defects or other identified genetic abnormalities, at any age over 21?   Yes ___   No ___ .

Name _____   Office Address _____

Office Phone _____ .

All responses will be treated as
HIGHLY CONFIDENTIAL MATERIAL.

Fifty-one questionnaires were mailed and 35 replies were received. Twenty-eight physicians indicated that they were willing to perform vasectomies as office procedures; five were not. One physician indicated a fee of $50.00, while eighteen would charge from $100.00—$125.00, and thirteen would charge from $150.00—$250.00. One urologist indicated that he would charge only what the patient was able to pay. Sixteen urologists would under no circumstances perform vasectomy on any man under the age of thirty-five. However, 27 would perform vasectomy on the single man over twenty-one, or a married man (his wife concurring) with a history of congenital defects or other identified genetic abnormalities. Only three urologists would perform vasectomy on men 20—25 years old without reservation, as would another three for men in the 26—30 age group.

Each answered questionnaire was subjected to close analysis. It was really quite remarkable how the standards of the responding urologists differed, making it difficult to categorize and classify these answers except as indicated above.

In connection with the development of the Planned Parenthood Center Vasectomy Clinic, the organizational structure and the logistical plans included an unpaid volunteer director, the regular nursing and volunteer staffs of the Center Clinic, a hired part-time orderly, and a physician staff of Texas-licensed urology residents in the late stages of their training. The latter were to be paid $25.00 per case out of the fee originally set for those who could pay it at $75.00. The patients who could not pay this fee, or any fee whatever, were not to be charged, although in each case, the resident was to receive the usual fee of $25.00. In addition, a graduate psychologist and a minister-social worker were employed for the purpose of screening all candidates. In doubtful cases, the physicians, or the Vasectomy Clinic Director made the final decisions.

The total amount of "seed money" was small and was generously provided by one of the Clinic's patrons. All instruments and supplies were furnished at cost by St. Luke's Episcopal Hospital.

The limitations of Clinic space made it necessary to operate the Vasectomy Clinic on a truncated Thursday night, starting at 6:30 P.M. because the Women's Clinic was operative until then, and on Friday evening, starting at 5:30 P.M. The cost of nursing care, that of the orderly, and other ancillary help was charged to the Vasectomy Clinic income. In effect, we started on a shoestring, and kept operating on a shoestring under less than ideal conditions.

After the instrument packs, the autoclave, and the supplies were all received, a newspaper item was released to the effect that the Vasectomy Clinic would begin operation in June 1970. This immediately precipitated a great rush of telephone inquiries, and it was apparent at once that the office staff could not begin to provide the information requested and still carry on its normal duties.

A detailed question-and-answer brochure, simply written and entitled "Vasectomy: An Effective Method of Birth Control" was therefore prepared which answered all of the questions from patients that could possibly be anticipated. On telephone inquiry, then, the prospective patient was asked for his name and address, and the brochure was mailed to him.

After the husband and his wife had studied the brochure and had made a positive decision, they then called the Clinic for an appointment for interview by the graduate psychologist and/or the minister-social worker. If the patient's income was in excess of what was considered low income, he was urged to see a private physician on the roster prepared earlier. As the reputation of the Clinic has increased, it has become increasingly difficult to turn many of these patients away.

If the patient was approved for vasectomy, the husband was given an instruction sheet, "What to Do in Preparing Yourself for Vasectomy" and both then signed the consent form (see below). An appointment for the surgery was then given. All questions with regard to the propriety of performing the vasectomy in less than clear-cut cases were referred to the physicians or to the Director for final decision. In all cases that were complicated by the presence of hernia, varicocele, or other scrotal pathology, referral to a private physician was insisted upon.

CONSENT FOR STERILIZATION OPERATION

WHEREAS the physicians of Planned Parenthood of Houston, Texas have been asked to perform an operation of sterilization on the undersigned husband, such an operation being known medically as a vas-ligation and section, and WHEREAS the physicians of Planned Parenthood of Houston are willing to perform said operation only upon the written consent and agreement of the undersigned husband and wife, freely and fully given, and WHEREAS the undersigned, by execution of this agreement, hereby give their consent and agreement, individually and jointly, to the performance of a vas-ligation and section upon the husband with the full understanding that said operation may forever and irrevocably deprive said husband of the ability to produce children or cause pregnancy in a female partner.

The undersigned further agree that neither Planned Parenthood of Houston nor physicians of Planned Parenthood of Houston shall be responsible in any way for any deleterious consequences resulting from said operation, and hereby release and discharge them from any or all claims and demands whatsoever which they, their heirs, executors, administrators, or assigns have or may have against Planned Parenthood of Houston by reason of any matter relative or incident to such operation.

We have read and fully understand all details of the brochure on "Vasectomy: An Effective Method of Birth Control" which was given to us by Planned Parenthood of Houston, and of which this consent form was an intrinsic part.

Signed this _____ day of _____, 19 _____

WITNESSES:

_____ (name)

                                            _____

                                                        (Husband)

_____ (address)

_____ (name)

                                            _____

                                                           (Wife)

_____ (address)

                                            _____

                                                       (Address)

Since the Vasectomy Clinic commenced operation, more than 900 vasectomies have been done, at a rate of about 40 each week. The average time now required for the performance of the operation varies from 8—15 minutes, depending on the individual surgeon and on certain anatomic characteristics. . . . As a usual rule, one resident can perform his allotted 7 to 8 vasectomies in about two hours.

The process of vasectomy has been simplified. We have learned to excise a liberal length of the vas which has been completely separated from its sheath, so that the tied ends, especially the proximal vas, may retract well into the sheath. Cotton ligature is used as the ties. It is not only one-tenth as expensive as chromic catgut, but produces much less tissue reaction. Still, we have learned that the tie must not be tied too tight, since it will then cut through the vas and enhance the chance of recanalization. We no longer use skin sutures; since the incisions are seldom more than one centimeter long, after the cut-tied ends of the vas are allowed to drop well into the depths of the scrotum, the walls of the incision coapt well. Necrosis of the skin edges, swelling, and the bleeding associated with the passage of the needle are avoided. This also avoids catching the vas and leaving it tied to the skin where it causes annoying discomfort. Release of the vas from the skin was subsequently done in three cases.

After the vasectomy has been completed, the orderly applies the dressing and the athletic supporter, the patient is given a printed "Instructions to Follow After Vasectomy," and he is dismissed after being given the surgeon's telephone number and name. Since most of the residents carry page "Bellboys," incident to their regular duties, they are easy to reach in the event of real or imagined urgency. In recent months, there has been a marked drop in the number of such calls from patients.

Complications have been few, but there have been complications. Scrotal hematoma, requiring hospitalization and evacuation occurred in two cases: the tenth and the twenty-fifth. Only the first offered the threat of malpractice harassment. On principle, however, we have elected to permit the patient's attorney to proceed with his threat of suit on the basis that the consent form is adequate protection against such legal action. One superficial abscess developed, requiring incision and drainage and a course of antibiotics. Recovery was uneventful, as it was in four additional cases of epididymitis. On the basis of lessons learned, none of these complications has occurred in the last 500 cases.

There have been five failures, two of which are classified as primary in that the subsequent semen checks were never free of sperm in large quantity at the six-week microscopic examination. In both cases, there was reason to believe that the vas had not been identified, both patients tolerating the procedure poorly. Since the vas segments are preserved in fixative, subsequent histologic study confirmed that only one vas had been removed. The semen specimens of three additional patients were negative at the six-week examination, but later became positive, resulting in two cases in pregnancies. These were shown to be frank cases of recanalization in that histologic examination of the specimens revealed vas segments for all cases. One patient had had a hydrocoele repair earlier, and the failure of the proximal segment of the vas to retract was attributed to the scarring of the earlier surgery.

We have considered it important to operate the Vasectomy Clinic in an atmosphere of good taste and high medical purpose. The continuing vigor of this Clinic reflects the cooperation and the approval of the medical community. Patients are being referred to the Clinic by former patients, by urologists, and by other physicians. A one-minute film strip discussing the usefulness of vasectomy was made and shown nightly at a late hour as a public service by television station KHTV. This stimulated considerable interest and suggests the potentially great value of similar public service strips on the national networks.

CONCLUSIONS

1. The Vasectomy Clinic of Houston's Planned Parenthood Center has demonstrated that large-scale clinics are feasible, practical, and fill a significant community need.

2. Such clinics are readily adaptable to large- and medium-

sized metropolitan centers containing one or more medical schools and medical centers which can provide the surgical manpower.

  3. A vasectomy clinic or a vasectomy referral service should be regarded as an intrinsic and important function of all Planned Parenthood Affiliates.

PLANNED PARENTHOOD OF HOUSTON VASECTOMY CLINIC

STATISTICAL ANALYSIS

AGE DISTRIBUTION

Age Range	Number	Percent	
21-26	134	15.5	Mean Age 32
27-32	339	39.4	Mode 29
33-38	226	26.3	
39-44	98	11.4	
45-50	43	5.0	
51-56	15	1.7	
56-60	5	0.6	
TOTALS	860	100%	

DURATION OF MARRIAGE

	Number	Percent	
Single	17	2.0	Mean 9.3
Less than one year	17	2.0	Mode 5.0
1-5	216	25.6	
6-10	323	38.3	
11-15	171	20.3	
16-20	63	7.4	
21-25	31	3.7	
26-30	6	0.7	
TOTALS	844	100%	

DISTRIBUTION — NUMBER OF CHILDREN PER FAMILY

	Number	Percent	
0-1	95	11.2	Mean 2.6
2-3	602	71.2	
4-5	127	15.0	
6-7	16	2.0	
8-10	5	0.6	
TOTALS	845	100%	

2   VASECTOMY IN A POPULATION CONTROL CENTER

by Lonny Myers, M.D.

Dr. Lonny Myers, an anesthesiologist married to a plastic surgeon, is a unique figure in the Midwest. An exuberant, relentless campaigner who has jabbed and goaded medical societies and all obstacles to fertility control for a dozen years, she started as a volunteer with Planned Parenthood, organized the Illinois Committee for Medical Control of Abortion in 1967, and became vice president of the National Association for Repeal of Abortion Laws, the coalition movement dedicated to the legalization of abortion as a feminine right. Convinced that population control is the paramount problem of our time, she helped found Chicago's Midwest Population Center, which houses contraceptive, abortion referral, and voluntary sterilization services under one roof.

In 1970, Dr. Myers gave up her regular medical practice, trained in vasectomy, and now runs one of the country's busiest vasectomy clinics at the Center. She is probably the only woman physician in the U.S. specializing in vasectomy.

For ten years (1959-1969), my interest in anesthesiology waned. My activities in the birth control movement had far more meaning for me. My life had three major divisions — anesthesiology/hospital, family, and "the movement." In the spring of 1969 I heard Paul Ehrlich of Zero Population Growth speak. The urgency hit me. I decided to shift my professional time to population.

In working with the birth control movement, it became clear to me that the major resistance to universal birth control was the need to use pregnancy as a punishment and use the fear of pregnancy as a means to control (however futile) sexual behavior. Our real obstruction was the refusal to allow people to express their sexuality without fear of evil consequences . . . and presenting pregnancy as an "evil consequence." I am committed to the promotion of pregnancy as a planned and joyful event, that must now be limited. We continue to force unwilling women to bear unwanted children because of our punitive attitudes toward genital sex. We have so many "wanted" babies because we teach and reward female sex role stereotypes — a fulfilled woman is one with many babies, etc. If we ceased to use pregnancy as punishment and ceased programming for parenthood, we might cease to have a population problem!

INADEQUACIES OF THE MEDICAL PROFESSION

The medical profession has chosen to kowtow to religion and tradition at the expense of the health of individual patients and the aggregate health of the nation. At maternal mortality meetings I have attended, abortion was not even mentioned. An entire session on illegitimacy did not even mention contraception, let alone the option for abortion. There was no plan to include contraception in all sex education courses or wherever reproduction is taught. I decided I wanted to get into sex education for medical students. Their lack of training was already recognized. I went to one of the medical schools where I had given speeches on occasion and spent several months discussing a program, talking with the dean and president. Assuming I would start in November, I did my last case (anesthesia) at Michael Reese Hospital on October 31, 1969. But the appointment never materialized.

I kept mulling over in my mind: population, sex education. How would I use my license to practice medicine? In February, the flash came: vasectomy! What other procedure demands a license, is simple to learn, and is desperately needed in the population movement? I started suggesting the idea to friends and colleagues. I got both positive and negative feedback. I met Dr. Joe Davis, president of AVS, whose support and encouragement were essential to my first step. He supervised the first vasectomy I performed on July 1, 1970. Had he ridiculed the idea or even discouraged me, I might not have gotten started.

THE NEED FOR A CLINIC

I knew I must work with a group in a clinic. I walked into Planned Parenthood unannounced and found Ben Lewis, the executive director. "What's new in abortion?" "But I'm not here about abortion. I want to do vasectomies." "Great," he replied enthusiastically. He called in staff personnel, and everyone was excited. I was elated. I vigorously continued my training, going back to New York to the Margaret Sanger Clinic several times; to the PP clinic in Milwaukee many times; to a general surgical clinic in Minneapolis where a surgeon does 20 vasectomies in three hours every Tuesday evening. But the medical advisory committee (consisting of male gynecologists, almost exclusively) decided against having me organize their vasectomy service. After all, what would that do to their reputation? A female anesthesiologist! (Incidentally, the public affairs committee voted in favor.) The last two weeks in July, I attended the postgraduate sex education course (for those interested in teaching in medical schools) at the Institute for Sex Research in Bloomington, Indiana (Kinsey's Institute). I was all the more convinced of the need to educate doctors. Even the course itself did not freely discuss some important behavior patterns.

The idea of doing vasectomies and using the money over and above expenses to support a sex/population program emerged. Many difficult but exciting discussions took place between me and the Reverend Don Shaw. Don had resigned from the Congress on Optimum Population and was available and very motivated to start something in this area. I provided creative energy, irritation, and confusion. Don worked furiously, organizing and making proposals for funding.

Since we have personal friends at *Playboy*, Don wrote and rewrote proposals, and our final plan was accepted by the Playboy Foundation, which resulted in an outright grant of $6,000 and a loan of $6,000. To this were added two personal loans of $1,000 each, and a $5,000 loan from AVS — a total of $19,000 as working capital. We hired a secretary who soon became a lot more than that. We found office space. We agonized over the composition of the corporation, deciding on a small one. The advisory board was "advised" that its purposes were to lend prestige, that they would not be involved in decision making, nor would they be solicited for money.

Recruitment of surgeons. Again many heated debates, but we agreed on the idea of selection on the basis of dedication to the cause. We sent a questionnaire to urologists, general surgeons, and obstetrician-gynecologists. We invited those interested in vasectomies to a luncheon meeting. In the meantime, I personally contacted all surgeons recommended by AVS in the Chicago area. From these two sources we came up with two urologists, three MD general surgeons, one osteopathic general surgeon, and me. We announced our opening in February 1971 with a big press conference in our not-yet-finished suite of rooms. We had appointed one of the urologists to be chief of clinical services. He was eloquent. We had post-vasectomy patients, including a Protestant minister and a senior editor of *Playboy*. Great coverage. We made the news in all three media. The next day — and few weeks — we went crazy with phone calls . . . information, but mainly appointments to sign up *now!* "I've been waiting for years," "You're great, just what we need!" As many as 40 calls in one day.

Don and I started doing all the interviewing ourselves. We developed a combination of group and individual interviews, opening with group instruction, then seeing each couple for a private interview. We reluctantly take the position of "devil's advocate." We pressure each candidate to envision himself in a new marriage, in love with someone who desperately wants to get pregnant. We push them into imagining a great tragedy affecting their wives and children. In fact, some applicants wonder which side we are on.

At first when I was doing a lot of the interviewing, everyone knew who Dr. Myers was. Later when we hired professional interviewers, some patients who signed up for Dr. Myers had quite a shock when I walked into the room. One black patient verbalized his anxiety about a woman operating on "that area." I asked him about his wife's doctor and went on about bias and prejudice — how can you keep expecting whites to deal with their prejudice and now not be willing to deal with yours? He began to loosen up and we joked a bit. By the time he decided it was okay, I told him it was all over and he could go home.

I am also the MD around to examine the patients. Some do a double take, but in general I have had no problems with the male/female angle. I am comfortable with myself and what I am doing. My training as an anesthesiologist makes me determined that no one should have pain, and the atmosphere is one of friendly conversation during the procedure. I insisted that we have a male technician and a male to prep the patient; I wanted to be very sure there were not just females in the operating room — ganging up, so to speak! Still, a few wives were startled when I came out and told them the operation was over.

VOLUNTARY STERILIZATION AND THE MEDICAL PROFESSION

The medical profession even today — not fifty years ago, not ten years ago, but *today* — refuses to inform the public about sterilization procedures. Of all the public health pamphlets that are proudly distributed by the AMA, not one describes either male or female sterilization. And believe me, it is not a matter of oversight. For at least five years and probably much longer, the suggestion of including vasectomies in their informational brochures has been repeatedly made and repeatedly turned down. The public is woefully ignorant, and this ignorance extends even to the medical profession. I had a doctor ask me, in all seriousness, if the volume of semen was reduced after vasectomy. There are doctors — graduates of our medical schools — with no idea of the anatomy or physiology of semen production. It is not a matter of forgetting — the subject is just not taught. I certainly was never taught the relationship of vasectomy to the production of semen.

The medical profession has traditionally perpetuated the glories of pronatalism, rejoicing at the birth of each infant. Doctors have done little or nothing to alter the myth that a woman with many children is somehow a "better" woman than the woman with one child or none at all. It is still prevalent to regard many children and many grandchildren as healthy and good.

We all grow. I am not demanding that the medical profession be clairvoyant; but I am saying that, as differentiated from any other area of medical care, attitudes toward sex and fertility control follow the public rather than lead it . . . and follow very slowly. In these times negligence in the area of birth control is not just a matter of injustice; it is a matter of human survival. We now face a population/environment crisis that demands a new approach to human sexuality and human reproduction.

The medical profession needs a mandate because it has been irresponsible and unscientific in its approach to human sexuality and fertility control, demonstrating little or no concern for the health of the individuals involved or the aggregate health of the nation.

A STATEMENT FROM THE MIDWEST POPULATION CENTER AND VASECTOMY CENTER OF CHICAGO

Those responsible for the vasectomy services of the Midwest Population Center regard the decision for vasectomy as a singularly important lifetime decision. We believe that grown men have the right to make the decision for vasectomy for themselves, as a basic matter of self-determination.

In view of overpopulation in the world, we regard a decision for vasectomy as demographically positive and responsible. Both the decision to have a child and the decision not to have a child should be the result of a serious and rational decision making process. We have been programmed by our culture, however, to be resigned and passive in the face of accidental and/or irresponsible parenthood and to be actively suspicious and scrupulously cautious about the decision to decline parenthood (or further parenthood). The Midwest Population Center affirms the seriousness and importance of both decisions and is pleased to serve those who, of their own free will and with full knowledge of the facts, elect permanent sterility. For this reason, any married male and any single or divorced male of 25 or over may apply for vasectomy at the Midwest Population Center. Single or divorced men under 25 years of age may be referred to a sympathetic private physician.

The Midwest Population Center staff of interviewers and physicians is party to the decision for vasectomy and, as such, shares responsibility in the decision making process. Our primary concern is that the decision for vasectomy be an informed one, fully voluntary and free of unwarranted expectations. To accomplish these purposes, those who apply for vasectomy at the Midwest Population Center are given group instruction and interviewed privately before acceptance for surgery.

I. The group instruction part of the interview hour is designed
    A. To set the tone of warmth, concern and good humor which characterizes our endeavor
    B. To share with our clients the facts about vasectomy as we perceive them
        1. The negative aspects, as indicated by that small percentage of vasectomized men who have regretted having had the surgery
            a. Later marriage; new wife desperately wants a baby
            b. Desire of children later in the same marriage
            c. Frustration that vasectomy did not remove sex hangups in themselves or their partners (an unwarranted expectation in any case)
        2. The positive aspects
            a. The achieving of desired sterility
            b. The enjoyment of sexual relations without fear of pregnancy
            c. The end of mechanical and/or chemical birth control techniques
        3. To review and clarify the preoperative and postoperative instructions
        4. To provide a realistic explanation of the surgical procedure
        5. To review and clarify the male reproductive system in relation to vasectomy surgery and consequent sterility

II. The private interview is designed
   A. To ascertain the extent to which the patient (and his wife) have thought through the decision
   B. To be sure that the man and his wife are mutually agreed on the procedure (no duress or unwarranted expectations, such as described in Paragraph III below)
   C. To ascertain psychological or medical problems that might contraindicate surgery at this time
   D. To deal with whatever personal questions are relevant

NOTE: The private interview is not designed for therapy or counseling in depth. It is expected that the vast majority of those seeking interviews will proceed with surgery. In those few cases where the decision appears questionable, the client should be told that his particular situation must be reviewed before proceeding further (i.e., scheduling surgery).

III. Special problem areas
   A. *Pregnancy.* If the client's wife is pregnant, it is important to determine whether or not the present pregnancy was planned and/or is definitely wanted. If the pregnancy is highly desired, the couple should be advised to proceed with vasectomy *only after the baby has arrived, is well, and at least one month old.* (There may be an occasional exception to this rule.)

   B. *Sexual Problems.* Men with sexual problems, such as impotence (failure to achieve erection), premature ejaculation, or unsatisfactory sexual performance, for whatever reasons, should be advised that *vasectomy will in no way help with these problems.* In most such instances, a statement to this effect should be added to the consent form to be signed by the man. Fear of pregnancy (though most always present) may in some cases be a rationalization for other sex hangups — especially in the female. This should be mentioned to clients when indicated, but it is not to be pressed or explored.

   C. *Medical Problems.* Medical problems that the interviewer feels should be reviewed before surgery should be noted on pink cards and clipped to the *outside* of the patient's folder.

D. *Psychological or Psychiatric Problems.* The Midwest Population Center has a Psychiatric Consultant who is available for special consultation. If the patient is in psychiatric therapy, the interviewer must be assured that the patient has discussed the possibility of vasectomy with his therapist. Permission must be given to consult with the therapist if necessary.

E. *Indecision.* In some cases, the interviewer may feel that the couple should have more time to think through the vasectomy decision. A second interview may be arranged for a month or two later (no further fee).

F. *Reversibility.* Clients who appear to have an emotional involvement in a reversible vasectomy are not good candidates for our vasectomy service. Patients should not be accepted for surgery unless they clearly intend permanent sterility, regardless of what the future holds for them. Those concerned with reversibility may be referred to private physicians via the Midwest Population Control staff.

3 SELECTING A MEDICAL FACILITY

by Lawrence Lader

The first step for any man seeking vasectomy is to get the advice of his own physician. The chances are that he will recommend a nearby clinic, general surgeon, or urologist doing vasectomy in his office. But since some physicians are still uninformed about vasectomy, the male applicant can easily contact the nearest clinic on his own. For a list of clinics by states, see Appendix I, page 256

If the applicant needs further help, he should write or phone the nearest Planned Parenthood office, listed in the telephone book of most major cities. If still unsatisfied, he can contact the Association for Voluntary Sterilization at 14 West 40 St., New York, N. Y. 10018 (Tel: 212-524-2344). AVS can advise on clinics or supply the name of one of its 1,600 cooperating physicians throughout the country.

The woman seeking voluntary sterilization should follow the same procedure, starting with her own physician or obstetrician-gynecologist. Since some hospitals still maintain the rigid and outdated obstacles of age-parity formulas and sterilization committees, a list of hospitals known to have progressive attitudes towards tubal ligations can be found in Appendix II, page 260

If a woman prefers laparoscopy or culdoscopy over the standard tubal ligation, a list of hospitals specializing in these techniques can be found in Appendix III, page 273, including a group performing them on an out-patient basis.

COST OF STERILIZATION AND POSSIBILITY OF INSURANCE COVERAGE

All surgeons' fees vary widely with the size of a city and the type of the physician's practice. As a general rule, however, the cost of vasectomy in a physician's office runs about $150, often including sperm tests and adjustable to the patient's need. Many clinics, like Planned Parenthood of Houston which charges $75, are specially geared to lower income brackets.

Price scales for female sterilization are more complicated. When a tubal ligation is performed shortly after childbirth, many physicians make no extra charge. Others add about $100 to the obstetrical fee. If performed at the time of caesarean section, some doctors make no extra charge, or a small charge. If the woman enters a hospital especially for sterilization, the fee should approximate any other simple abdominal procedure — around $250, depending on the patient's means and whether she has semiprivate or private accommodations. Laparoscopy and culdoscopy are too new for a firm price scale, but run about $200-$300 for a private patient.

In many states, Blue Cross-Blue Shield and Medicaid insurance cover all or part of the costs of voluntary sterilization. For a chart outlining the scope of this coverage, see Appendix IV, page 278. Some private medical insurance policies also provide coverage. In each case the applicant should contact the nearest agency handling his insurance coverage.

The most recent financial assistance for voluntary sterilization comes from the U. S. Government's Office of Economic Opportunity. In a letter dated June 15, 1971, to the Association for Voluntary Sterilization, Dr. George Contis, Director of OEO's Family Planning Program, Office of Health Affairs, stated: "On May 18, the Community Action Memo 37-A was amended to permit the use of OEO grant funds for surgical procedures intended to result in sterilization."

Part Nine ♀♂

The Legal Right to Voluntary Sterilization for the Applicant and Physician

1 KNOW YOUR RIGHTS ABOUT VOLUNTARY STERILIZATION

by Harriet F. Pilpel, AVS legal counsel

VOLUNTARY STERILIZATION LEGAL

Voluntary sterilization is legal in all 50 states. Only one — Utah — limits *the reasons* for which voluntary sterilization may be performed. In Utah, the operation may be performed only for "medical necessity," which means for both therapeutic and eugenic reasons. Utah is presently considering repeal of this law, and in 1969 Connecticut repealed a similar law, the repeal becoming effective October 1971.

Three states, Georgia, North Carolina, and Virginia, have recently passed laws setting forth specific conditions to be complied with by those who choose voluntary sterilization (consultation, consent of spouse, age of patient, etc.), but voluntary sterilization for all reasons is legal in these states.

Voluntary sterilization is one important method of birth control. It is the best method for those who have decided they should not have or do not want to have any more children.

Not only is it legal in all states, but the American Medical Association stated in 1961 that sterilization poses no greater danger of civil liability than any other medical and surgical procedures. (Medicolegal Forms with Legal Analysis, Chicago: Law Department, American Medical Association, 1961, p. 28.) In May 1968, an editorial in the *Journal of the American Medical Association* (May 27, 1968, Vol. 204, p. 209) reiterated this view, stating (after referring to the special situation in Connecticut and Utah) that "Contraceptive sterilization is nowhere forbidden in this country," and that "Voluntary sterilization of man is safe, quick, effective, and legal."

The Joint Commission on Accreditation of Hospitals has taken an explicitly permissive position on voluntary sterilization. Hospitals are free to make their own rules on this matter.

In 1969, the American College of Obstetricians and Gynecologists revised its Standards applicable to voluntary sterilization. These Standards previously recommended a formula based on the woman's age and the number of children as the criterion for the performance of a requested sterilization. This age-parity formula has been deleted entirely. The new ACOG Standards now say, after referring to the "many states [that] have no statutes on sterilization," that it "can be performed on anyone who is legally capable of giving the obstetrician-gynecologist permission to operate upon her.... Regardless of state laws, however, each hospital must establish its own regulations concerning sterilization.... These should be developed by the members of the department of obstetrics and gynecology and approved by the medical staff and appropriate governing body...."

PHYSICIAN'S LEGAL RESPONSIBILITY FOR VOLUNTARY STERILIZATION SAME AS FOR OTHER SURGICAL PROCEDURES

As with any other surgical procedure, the consent of the patient should be obtained in writing for a voluntary sterilization operation, and the patient should be advised not only as to the nature of the operation but also of the fact that its success is not guaranteed, i.e., that in rare instances sterility may not result from such an operation.

Generally speaking, therefore, if this basic requirement is complied with, the physician has the legal right to perform a voluntary sterilization operation and no liability will follow. The only exception is, as with other surgical procedures, if the operation is performed in a negligent manner. (At the American Urological Association meeting in May 1965, it was announced that there is now available a malpractice liability insurance policy which includes voluntary sterilization with coverage up to $1,000,000 for any doctor involved in a damage suit.)

We know of no successful action for damages against a physician based upon the non-negligent performance of a voluntary sterilization operation where the informed consent of the patient had been obtained; and we know of no prosecution in any state against a physician for performing a voluntary sterilization operation. It is sometimes said that physicians may be charged with "mayhem" if they perform a voluntary sterilization operation, even with the consent of the patient. We are satisfied that this is not so. Originally, mayhem in a bygone era meant the wilful infliction of injury on oneself or another which interfered with the injured person's ability to bear arms for the king. For many technical as well as common sense reasons we believe, and a recent case in California so held, that there is no basis for any fear or doubt along these lines.

A WORD WITH RESPECT TO MINORS AND INCOMPETENT PERSONS

Minors may be deemed not capable of giving legally effective consent to a sterilization (or any other) operation. Also, an incompetent person may not understand the nature and consequences of the operation and may not be competent to consent to its performance. In cases of minors and incompetents, special precautions should be taken (as with any other medical or surgical matter) and the family and the physician should consult attorneys familiar with these matters in their own state as to how to proceed.

VOLUNTARY STERILIZATION NOT ONLY LEGAL BUT IMPORTANT FOR PUBLIC POLICY TODAY

Various Federal governmental agencies such as the Agency for International Development, the Department of Health, Education and Welfare, and the Department of Defense have considered voluntary sterilization as an aspect of family planning which should be available for an informed decision by the individual in accordance with sound medical practice.

Under the 1967 amendments to Title IV of the Social Security Act (Aid to Families with Dependent Children) and Title V (Maternal and Child Health Programs), state and local welfare agencies are required, as a condition of state plan approval, to provide family planning services for each child, relative, and other essential person in the home without regard to marital status or age.

The objective of these amendments, according to former Secretary of Health, Education and Welfare, John Gardner, is to offer such services so as to reduce the incidence of out-of-wedlock birth and to otherwise strengthen family life.

VOLUNTARY STERILIZATION COVERED BY MEDICAID AND INSURANCE

According to the most recent survey by AVS, the Federal/State Medicaid program, in which the Federal government contributes to State Medicaid funds, now operates in 39 states. Of these, 34 states, plus the District of Columbia and the Virgin Islands, report that they pay for voluntary sterilization under Medicaid. The majority of these states do not report making any distinction regarding the reasons for which the operation is performed.

Blue Cross and Blue Shield insurance companies pay for voluntary sterilization in most states across the country. Of Blue Cross groups replying to AVS from 44 states, 40 plus the District of Columbia reported paying hospital expenses for voluntary sterilization done for "medical necessity," and 35 plus the District of Columbia reported paying for those done for socio-economic reasons as well.

Of Blue Shield organizations replying from 47 states, 39 plus the District of Columbia (and some state of Washington plans) reported paying for the operation for "medical reasons"; and 33, plus the District of Columbia (and some state of Washington plans), for "socio-economic reasons."

VOLUNTARY STERILIZATION AS A HEALTH MEASURE

Voluntary sterilization, in addition to being a contraceptive method, can also be a health measure.

In May of 1965, the New York Academy of Medicine formally adopted the definition of health previously adopted by the World Health Organization, to wit: "Health is a state of complete physical, mental and social well-being and not merely the absence of disease or infirmity."

Psychiatrist Robert W. Laidlaw and Medora S. Bass, M.A., in their article, "Voluntary Sterilization as It Relates to Mental Health," state: "Voluntary sterilization can and does contribute to mental health... by reducing the anxiety caused by fear of unwanted pregnancies; by preventing children from being born to irresponsible parents with resultant neglect and social ills.... All this can be accomplished without unfavorable psychological effects and with a high ratio of satisfaction." Postoperative follow-up studies on both men and women, according to the Laidlaw-Bass article, indicate ratios of satisfaction in the area of 94% and 96%.

Of course, there are also many physical conditions which in the opinion of physicians require voluntary sterilization operations.

VOLUNTARY — NOT COMPULSORY

We are concerned with *voluntary* sterilization. *Voluntary* sterilization is not to be confused with *compulsory* sterilization. About three-fifths of the states today provide for compulsory sterilization in some circumstances. One of the early *compulsory* sterilization statutes — a Virginia statute — was challenged as unconstitutional. The case finally got to the United States Supreme Court. It involved the sterilization of a woman

in a public institution in Virginia whose feeble-minded
mother was in the same institution and who had already given
birth to a feeble-minded child. In this case — *Buck vs. Bell* —
Justice Oliver Wendell Holmes, Jr. wrote the opinion of the
Court sustaining the statute — uttering the now famous words,
"Three generations of imbeciles are enough." Some years
later an Oklahoma compulsory sterilization statute was challenged in a case that also reached the United States Supreme
Court. The Court, without overruling *Buck vs. Bell,* declared
it unconstitutional on equal protection grounds. Recent United
States Supreme Court decisions in related areas suggest that
today all the *compulsory* statutes may be constitutionally vulnerable.
It is clear that a statute making *voluntary* sterilization available
is constitutional and is indeed in aid of constitutional rights.
It is equally clear that a statute affirmatively acknowledging
voluntary sterilization is not needed in order to make it lawful.

Part Ten ☿♂

Overcoming Obstructions to Voluntary Sterilization

1   VOLUNTARY STERILIZATION AND THE MEDICAL PROFESSION

by Helen Edey, M.D.

Despite the soaring rate of voluntary sterilization in the U.S. — an estimated 1 million in 1971 — these operations have been performed by a somewhat limited group of physicians, hospitals, and clinics, and the medical profession as a whole still maintains many barriers against the procedure. The following articles examine such negative policies, particularly among urologists and hospitals, and point up the necessity of a sweeping revision of attitudes.

There are two reasons why physicians should be well informed about all methods of contraception. (1) It has been agreed that there are damaging psychologic and social consequences to the mother, to her family, and to the child she bears when it is unwanted. (2) Most physicians, biologists, sociologists, ecologists, and politicians, including President Nixon, have realized that it will be necessary to encourage people to want small families.

But many physicians appear rather ambivalent about the matter. It is my thesis that voluntary sterilization, as a method of family planning, is not generally considered rationally on its merits. It should be thoroughly considered whenever a person is sure that he or she never wants any more children.

The high failure rates of other methods are often not appreciated. The annual failure rates sound reassuringly low, but if a mechanical method is used for a period of fifteen years, there is a greater than 50 per cent chance of having another child. Even if an intrauterine device is successfully retained, there is a 15 per cent risk of pregnancy in ten years. Every physician knows about the current fears concerning the pill. Many couples are continuously fearful of pregnancy. A physician who does not offer the option of sterilization is saying, in effect, "you must continue to take these chances."

It is true that with voluntary sterilization there is the chance of regret, in less than 2 per cent of cases according to many surveys, but is it up to the physician to decide which chance the patient must take? If his own religion or convictions prevent him from considering this option with the patient, he should refer the patient elsewhere, as is now recommended in abortion cases.

At present only a minority of urologists will perform vasectomies. Some even tell their patients that it is illegal. Many say that they fear lawsuits, although, as the counsel of the AMA has stated, there is no more risk of a malpractice suit with this operation than with any other. No suit against a physician or hospital has ever been won when the operation has been competently performed and informed consent has been obtained. Fears about psychologic complications are exaggerated; they are rare. In the most recent large study, that of the Simon Population Trust in England, which reported in 1969 on more than 1,000 vasectomies, the patients' sexual life improved in 73.1 per cent of cases, deteriorated in 1.5 per cent and remained the same in the rest.

A man or woman of means, sophistication, and persistence can shop around for a physician and hospital with relatively liberal criteria. But if a person is restricted by financial or geographic limitations, or has little information, he or she often has no opportunity to consider the pros and cons of voluntary sterilization.

A survey has just been made by the Association for Voluntary Sterilization of the 22 hospitals in Nassau and Suffolk Counties (New York) that have obstetric services. Information has been obtained from 20. Only one hospital in either county states that it will do a sterilization on a woman under thirty years old with fewer than five children! Several will never do a sterilization except for medical indications, and some of these are not Catholic hospitals. Why won't they? Committees and regulations have been declared unnecessary by the American College of Obstetricians and Gynecologists. In August 1970, they further stated: "If sterilization is requested by the patient, and her physician agrees, consultation is not necessary." Many hospitals ignore these guidelines. What has happened to the alleged freedom of a woman to decide not to have any more unwanted children?

A study of sterilization services and policies in 372 teaching hospitals in the United States and Canada has just been completed by the Center for Population Planning of the University of Michigan. I quote from some of their conclusions:

Many hospitals had policies against performing voluntary sterilizations for men or referring them for operations in the private offices of urologists, despite the fact that vasectomy is a much simpler operation than tubal ligation.

No consistent medical practice existed regarding voluntary sterilization and consequently there had been no valid reason for refusal of many applications.

Eligibility requirements in the types of hospitals covered varied so widely as to make it clear that arbitrary value systems, not scientifically based rules, were in use.

A study was made in the summer of 1970 for the New York City Department of Health of policies and practices in local hospitals. Examples of the ratio of sterilizations to deliveries in non-Catholic hospitals in 1969 ranged from lows of 3 in 2,510 deliveries and 68 per 4,854 in hospitals with restrictive policies to highs of 276 per 1,915 and 420 per 2,402 in hospitals with more liberal policies. The latter have waiting lists. Vasectomies were hardly ever performed.

The assumption of the right to specify the family size of the patient by hospital is now being challenged in court. Hospitals are arbitrarily determining the fertility of others whenever they withhold crucial information and services. I, therefore, urge that there no longer be sterilization committees or regulations which interfere with the doctor-patient relationship, or with the right of the physician to practice medicine as he thinks best. I further urge each physician to consider without prejudice the wish of a patient to terminate his or her fertility, even though the physician might not choose it for himself in similar circumstances. There are certainly contraindications to voluntary sterilization, but not having enough children to meet some arbitrary number should not be one of them.

2   VOLUNTARY MALE STERILIZATION: AN EDITORIAL

Journal of the American Medical Association (May 27, 1968, Vol. 204, No. 9)

The critical breakthrough in the traditional policy of obstruction by influential medical organizations came in 1968 with an editorial in the Journal of the American Medical Association. Then in 1969, the American College of Obstetricians and Gynecologists abandoned its old age-parity hurdles and approved female sterilization at the request of the patient.

Voluntary sterilization of man is safe, quick, effective, and legal. Yet physicians are reluctant to use the procedure, even though it seems to offer the ideal contraceptive for a husband when his family has become as large as he and his wife want or can afford. Why do these men, particularly if they are in the lower income portion of the population, have so much difficulty obtaining a sterilization operation?

Physicians offer many reasons. One is religion. The Roman Catholic hierarchy forbids male sterilization as a contraceptive method. Obviously, the Catholic physician and the Catholic patient must resolve any medico-religious conflicts in accord with their own consciences and beliefs. But the rest of the country must not be deprived of a legitimate method of contraception because of the opposition of any outside group.

A serious concern to physicians is the legality of voluntary sterilization. There are four varieties of sterilization: eugenic, punitive, therapeutic, and contraceptive. The first two do not fall within the definition of voluntary sterilization. There are no legal bars to therapeutic sterilization in any state, except that Utah has a statute requiring "reasons of medical necessity." Excluding this state, contraceptive sterilization is nowhere forbidden in this country. Georgia has passed a law which assures immunity from criminal or civil suits (excluding of course, negligent performance) for physicians who perform voluntary sterilization. This law clearly legalizes voluntary sterilization in that state. North Carolina and Virginia have similar laws. But voluntary sterilization is *not* illegal in states *lacking* a statute similar to Georgia's. Gampell[1] points out that most states have a general provision that "no act or omission is criminal or punishable except as prescribed or authorized by the appropriate code. It is an equally well recognized rule of law that penal statutes must be construed to reach no further than their words and that no one can be made subject to them by implication." Fundamentally, then, voluntary sterilization is legal in all 50 states (although limited to "medical necessity" in Utah).

A related concern is that of civil damages. The American Medical Association stated in 1961 that sterilization poses no greater danger of liability than other medical and surgical procedures alleged to have been negligently performed.[2] This opinion remains valid today.

Sterilization of a man is an extremely simple operation. Usually it can be done in the physician's office, using local anesthetic. The patient need lose little or no time from work. In psychologically stable patients the operation does not impede erection or ejaculation; sexual potency is unaltered. After vasectomy the physician should insist that his patient have seminal analysis to ensure that the operation has been successful; if the ejaculate contains no sperm six months to a year after vasectomy, sterilization is presumably complete.

This completeness has seemed to be another factor limiting the more widespread use of vasectomy for contraception. Obviously the technique is not the ideal method of contracep-

tion for a man who hopes to father children at a later date.
But for those who have a family and wish to limit its size,
vasectomy is a highly satisfactory method. Nevertheless, circumstances do arise which might lead the vasectomized man to
desire his lost fertility. Thus it is important to note that
plastic surgery has been successful in repairing vasectomies in
50% to 90% of cases (see, for example, Dorsey,[3] reporting 18
successful operations out of 20 attempts, and Roland,[4] with 7
out of 9).

In the past, some psychiatrists and urologists argued
against the procedure because of alleged psychiatric trauma.
Although follow-up studies indicate mostly favorable results, a
few serious problems have been reported; but Ferber et al.,[5]
suggest that, in many instances in which sexual and psychological pathology is attributed to an antecedent vasectomy,
there was in fact evidence of psychiatric disorder before the
vasectomy was performed. Some of the "bad" results occurred
in "men who chose the operation for clearly symbolic and self-
mutilative reasons." It should be possible to identify most such
individuals beforehand.

In the patients studied by Ferber et al., subjectively
unsatisfactory results occurred in 3 of 73 patients (72 of the
73 would have the vasectomy performed again if they had it
to do over); each of these three men had a preexisting potency
difficulty. The strongest contraindication to vasectomy, in the
opinion of Ferber et al., was disagreement between husband and
wife over its advisability. This opinion seems strongly supported
by common sense.

There are, then, some contraindications of varying
relevancy. Perhaps the following can serve as preliminary
guidelines, subject to change as experience accumulates: if
a man can reconcile the operation with his religion; if he has
several children; if he lacks observable psychiatric sex-oriented
stigmata; and if his wife agrees to the operation — surely, then,
he should be able to obtain a vasectomy for reasons of contraception alone.

1. Gampell, R. J.: Legal Status of Therapeutic Abortion and Sterilization in the United States, *Clin Obstet Gynec* 7:22-36 (March) 1964.

2. *Medicolegal Forms with Legal Analysis,* Chicago: Law Department, American Medical Association, 1961, p. 28.

3. Dorsey, J. W.: Surgical Correction of Postvasectomy Sterility, *J Int Coll Surg* 27:453-456 (April) 1957.

4. Roland, S. I.: Splinted and Non-splinted Vasovasotomy, *Fertil Steril* 12:191-195 (March-April) 1961.

5. Ferber, A. S. Tietze, C.; and Lewit, S.: Men with Vasectomies: A Study of Medical, Sexual, and Psychosocial Changes, *Psychosom Med* 29: 354-366 (July-Aug) 1967.

3   CHANGES IN MANUAL OF STANDARDS FOR OBSTETRIC-GYNECOLOGIC HOSPITAL SERVICES

American College of Obstetricians and Gynecologists

The 1969 edition of "Standards for Obstetric-Gynecologic Hospital Services," the publication of the American College of Obstetricians and Gynecologists which is widely accepted by the medical profession as a guideline and set of standards, contains a significant change from preceding issues on the subject of voluntary sterilization. Previously, in regard to the female sterilization operation, ACOG guidelines mentioned a certain number of children together with a certain age of the mother as a criterion for a hospital's providing her with a requested sterilization. In the latest edition, this age-parity formula has been deleted entirely. The section on "Surgical Sterilization" on page 54 now states:

REVISION APPROVED BY THE ACOG EXECUTIVE BOARD, AUGUST 1970

"If an operation to accomplish sterilization is recommended by the physician for medical indications, the recorded opinion of a knowledgeable consultant should be obtained.

"If sterilization is requested by the patient, and her physician agrees, consultation is not necessary. (Emphasis by Ed.)

"In all cases where sterilization is performed primarily or results from an indicated operation, it is important that the patient understand that restoration of fertility is unlikely."

4 THE FUTURE SCOPE OF COURT ACTION

by Jeremiah S. Gutman

Now that abortion statutes and individual applications by patients to secure desired abortions have become almost everyday subjects of litigation, comparable issues on sterilization are beginning to find their ways into the courts. For too long have the mores and values of some been dignified and codified so as to become the involuntary limitations upon the freedom of others. Whether the arguments be of constitutional dimension or lesser in scope, whether the hospitals involved be publicly owned and operated or completely private or even parochial (or somewhere in between), courts all over the country are finding lawsuits being filed to compel the performance of requested procedures. No effort of which I am aware is being made to force any physician to perform a procedure which he regards as medically unsound, ethically improper, or personally distasteful. The thrust is against the institutions of society to require them to find willing personnel for those entitled to medical service from the State, and against hospitals themselves to make facilities available to physicians who wish to perform the procedures.

Experience so far has been both satisfying and frustrating. The satisfaction arises from the repeated prompt performance of the surgical procedure upon the commencing of a lawsuit. The frustration arises from the unwillingness of institutions to litigate and test the issues and provide the precedents which will lead to wider scale reforms and liberalization. The demand is increasing. The condition of the nation and the world, as well as the rising awareness of the indignity inherent in being unable to control one's body and its functions, all will inevitably lead to the removal of the presently widespread legal and practical obstacles to ready availability of sterilization procedures. It is reasonable to predict that within the next year or two any adult will be able readily and inexpensively to procure a sterilization.

5 "OPERATION LAWSUIT"

by John R. Rague

Notwithstanding the tremendous increase in popularity of voluntary sterilization within the past few years, innumerable women across the country are still being denied sterilization operations they need and want because of archaic and restrictive hospital regulations. Although many hospitals have modernized their rules and now follow the guidelines of the American College of Obstetricians and Gynecologists, which state: "...[Voluntary sterilization] can be performed on anyone who is legally capable of giving the obstetrician-gynecologist permission to operate upon her...," too many other hospitals still retain outmoded age-parity formulas and irrational restrictions on an operation which should be readily available to all adults who seek it. Some hospitals, for example, still require that a woman be 35 years old and have 5 children before the "Sterilization and Abortion Committee" of the hospital will seriously consider her request for the operation. In these times this is as out of place as witch hunts and voodoo.

All methods of birth control, including voluntary sterilization, should be not only readily available, but also *paid for* by the state in the case of the medically indigent. A step in this direction was taken recently when the Office of Economic Opportunity decided at long last to allow OEO funds to be used to pay for voluntary sterilizations in local family planning programs. However, any recalcitrant hospital with a Catholic-influenced sterilization committee and a pro-natalist philosophy is still a formidable roadblock to, and a destructive influence on, rational and humane practices in providing needed birth control services to the public.

Consequently, the Association for Voluntary Sterilization (AVS) has, within the past two years, aided several women who desired sterilization but who had been refused it by their local hospitals. Mrs. Janet Stein of Mohegan Lake, New York, sued the Northern Westchester Hospital in Mount Kisco both to obtain the operation and to force a liberalization of the hospital's rules. Backed by AVS and the New York Civil Liberties Union, she succeeded. Mrs. Paska Ivezaj of the Bronx, New York, similarly sued Fordham Hospital in the Bronx, one of the most intransigent hospitals known to AVS in regard to voluntary sterilization. (There had been an "unwritten rule" that *no* voluntary sterilizations were to be performed at Fordham for *any* reason.) Mrs. Ivezaj also obtained her operation as a result of the lawsuit, and Fordham reportedly has also liberalized its regulations.

Other lawsuits are in progress in Michigan, Massachusetts, and other states — all aimed at forcing hospitals to provide adequate, needed, and requested birth control services (sterilization) free from sectarian influence and antiquated pronatalist policies. To broaden this trend and to capitalize on the increasing willingness of women to refuse to take "no" for an answer, AVS decided to formalize an effort at persuading hospitals to mend their ways. Dubbed "Operation Lawsuit," the project brings together Zero Population Growth, Inc., and the American Civil Liberties Union with AVS in a new alliance to carry out a simple plan — to find and help women in local communities who have been denied sterilization, to obtain cooperation of local ACLU attorneys, and — if all efforts at persuasion of the hospital fail — to sue the hospital in order to 1) obtain the requested sterilization, 2) liberalize the hospital regulations to make the operation freely available, and 3) obtain payment for damages commensurate with injuries incurred.

Mrs. Shirley Radl, Executive Director of ZPG, wrote a "kickoff" letter to all ZPG chapters stating the importance of this project in the national ZPG effort to stabilize America's population growth. AVS sent with this letter a complete Information Kit on the project. Edward J. Ennis, Chairman of the ACLU, sent out an Information Sheet to ACLU affiliates across the country. Mrs. Radl then made personal visits and/or phone calls to 20 selected ZPG chapters. Many responded affirmatively to this project and are in process of finding a woman who wants to make the test case needed in her community.

AVS has made its Field Director, Courtland Hastings, available to all ZPG chapters for guidance and help on "Operation Lawsuit." AVS feels that if enough hospitals across the country find themselves facing lawsuits by women, including demands for damages incurred as a result of the hospital's refusal to provide the operation, hospital policies in general may soon be brought into the 20th century. As NYCLU attorney Jeremiah Gutman has said, hospitals are on very dubious constitutional grounds when they refuse sterilization to a woman who is sure she wants no more children and requests that permanent and reliable birth control be provided her. To insure that it is provided is the goal of "Operation Lawsuit."

6   POPULATION CRISIS RESOLUTION

United Methodist Church

Except for the Roman Catholic Church and some Orthodox Jewish groups, almost all Protestant, Jewish and other denominations support the ethical and religious basis of voluntary sterilization. Rabbi Balfour Brickner, for example, Director of the Commission on Interfaith Activities, Union of American Hebrew Congregations, states, "Voluntary sterilization is a significant and valuable method of birth control for those couples who have completed their families and are sure they want no more children."

Perhaps the most comprehensive Protestant statement on sterilization and all forms of birth control has come from the Methodist Church.

The population explosion brought on by medical and technological advances in the prolonging of life poses for man an unprecedented threat. The strong possibility of mass starvation looms ahead in some nations, with its concomitant of social upheaval. The rapid depletion of natural resources faces many countries.

The quality of our lives is increasingly threatened as runaway population growth places staggering burdens upon societies unable to solve even their present growth problems.

The population explosion threatens rich and poor nations alike. Poor nations find themselves on a treadmill of misery as their population growth offsets to a considerable extent their economic growth. Several affluent nations, like the U.S., though growing more slowly, will still double their population every sixty to eighty years, if present growth rates continue.

A full-scale effort must be made to stem the flood. Therefore, we urge the following action:

BY THE CHURCH

1. That the church recognize rapid population growth to be a matter of great religious and moral concern, producing a pressure of numbers that makes the problems of human society almost unmanageable, and threatening to alter the environment that sustains all life.

2. That the church devise education programs that will alert its constituencies and the general public to the fact and the nature of the population problem and the dangers it holds for man if left unmet.

3. That the church provide action programs that will help produce the changes in public policies and attitudes necessary for society to embark on new, creative, and vigorous efforts to stop the population explosion.

4. That the various denominations and the National Council of Churches and the World Council of Churches provide assistance and leadership to their constituencies in helping meet the population crisis.

5. That the church lay a moral responsibility upon the leaders of government and society to undertake a maximum and sustained effort to meet the population crisis, employing whatever funds and personnel and creating whatever agencies are necessary for that purpose. Special appeals should be made to charitable foundations to assume responsibility for programs devoted to this issue.

6. That the church underscore the moral necessity of adopting the small family norm as an essential principle for stabilizing the size of the population, and thus protecting the quality of life.

7. That church-related hospitals take the lead in eliminating those hospital administrative restrictions on voluntary sterilization and abortion which exceed the legal requirements in their respective political jurisdictions, and which frustrate the intent of the law where the law is designed to make the decision for sterilization and abortion largely or solely

the responsibility of the person most concerned.

8. That church agencies structure family planning skills and services into the training of missionary personnel, into medical programs and institutions, and into development programs, and that such family planning services be integrated as much as is possible with other family planning programs in host countries.

BY THE GOVERNMENT

1. That national governments create major agencies to deal solely with the population crisis. The development of atomic energy and the reaching of the moon took place only because major agencies were created solely for those purposes, told to achieve those objectives as soon as humanly possible, and given the money and manpower needed for the task.

Action at least as bold and massive will be required to stem the population crisis, a crisis which presents problems more complex than those of either the atom or of space.

2. That national legislative bodies create special committees on population, said committees to be responsible for assisting them discharge their responsibility effectively, as they seek to meet the population crisis.

That the U.S. Congress create either a Joint Select Committee on Population or that each of the two houses in Congress create its own Select Committee on Population, said committee(s) to be responsible for assisting Congress in meeting the population crisis, and to be financed and staffed adequately for their purpose.

3. That nations offer to share with each other the advances in technology, the experience in effective programming, and the material resources that would be helpful in carrying out family planning and population policies.

That maximum feasible assistance be given to all other nations in meeting their population growth problem, with full support also for international population efforts, such as those of the United Nations and the International Planned Parenthood Federation.

4. That states remove the regulation of abortion from the criminal code, placing it instead under regulations relating to other procedures of standard medical practice. Abortion would be available only upon request of the person most directly concerned.

5. That the remaining legal and administrative restrictions on voluntary sterilization be removed and that the individual after counseling be given the right to decide concerning his or her own sterilization.

BY THE INDIVIDUAL

1. That he recognize the moral dimensions of the population crisis, which poses such grave consequences for the future of man, and accept as his duty the responsibility for helping end this growing threat to the quality and existence of human life.

2. That, in planning their family, a couple should recognize that families with more that two children contribute to the population explosion.

3. That he encourage his church and government leaders to act with the boldness and vigor needed to meet this population crisis.

CONCLUSION

Since the population problem is so acute, imaginative and vigorous action is required on a grand scale. Let us, therefore, act now, that children may not be born to suffer and to experience despair, but rather may be the blessed fruit of love and the hope of a good tomorrow.

Conclusion

THE FUTURE OF VOLUNTARY STERILIZATION

by Lawrence Lader

The national groundswell towards voluntary sterilization, as the *Chicago Tribune* reported recently, "has taken the medical profession completely by surprise."[1] Not only has public demand, stimulated for decades by a relatively small organization like AVS and more recently by Planned Parenthood, run far ahead of the policies and facilities of organized medicine and governmental health agencies; but even today most doctors have just come to accept a medical procedure never barred by any state law. In fact, the main obstacle to the increasing impact of voluntary sterilization on family planning remains the apathy and obstructions of medical and governmental policy.

A significant case in point is the frustrations of Puerto Rican women living in New York's Spanish Harlem. Female sterilization has long been a popular form of birth control in Puerto Rico itself, easily available despite the opposition of the Roman Catholic Church. Yet in its 1970 research report on Harlem, Columbia University's International Institute for the Study of Human Reproduction concluded, "There is a demand for sterilization, particularly from Puerto Ricans, which is poorly met at present." Noting that "sterilization is not advocated in New York City nor is it easily obtainable," the researchers found that many Puerto Rican women "complained of the difficulty of getting the operation in New York" and "felt the positions of hospitals and doctors were unreasonable."

The most frequent obstacles were expense and that the applicant had too few children. One woman was told sterilization could never be done in the United States unless her life was in danger; two others that it was prohibited no matter how many children they had. Despite the "relatively high proportion of sterilized women," the researchers found, ironically enough, that 23 per cent of the sample had been sterilized while living in Puerto Rico, and 18 per cent had traveled from New York to Puerto Rico to be sterilized.[2]

"Why has the American Medical Association chosen *not* to publish information regarding sterilization even though millions are ignorant of this safe, permanent method of birth control?" asks Dr. Lonny Myers. The basic policy of the profession, unfortunately, has always been pro-natalist — the glorification of large families and rampant fertility, with little concern over personal or social damage from unwanted children. Organized medicine has failed to educate either the public or its own students at medical schools. "I have personally attended so-called scientific sessions where the management of teenage pregnancies and post-delivery counseling was discussed without even mentioning contraception, let alone voluntary sterilization and abortion," adds Dr. Myers. It was not until 1971 that a New York medical school established a student course on the political and social aspects of abortion, probably the first in the nation. No similar course has been started on sterilization.

These policies stem not only from old-fogeyism but an ingrained subservience to political and religious pressure groups. Hypocritically, the medical profession pays no heed to the medico-religious beliefs of Christian Scientists or Jehovah's Witnesses, whose membership is too limited. But the birth control, sterilization, and abortion prohibitions of the Catholic Church and some fundamentalist Protestants easily bludgeon many doctors into inaction.

The crowning failure has been to ignore the population crisis. "Our shirked responsibility in not having pushed population control soon enough," as Dr. Edmund Overstreet, professor

of obstetrics and gynecology at the University of California
School of Medicine, San Francisco, calls it.[3] Despite evidence
that world population will double from 3½ to 7 billions at present
growth rates by the year 2000, and that the U. S. population of
151 millions in 1950 may at least double by the end of the century, medical societies have ignored the danger of ecological
disaster. They remain equally aloof from the achievement of a
stabilized population, certainly a national health priority; and
from the only possible method of reaching it: the acceptance by
every family of a limit of two children. Although the "Stop at
Two" movement has gained broad national support recently,
no medical society — the agency best equipped to reach the public — has even passed a resolution of approval.

   Particularly distressing is the failure of physicians to educate the middle class, that group which makes up the bulk of
their patients and accounts for almost 70 per cent of all births.
This failure is borne out by a recent study of over 1,000 faculty
and students at Cornell University, a reasonable sample of the
educated middle class. Only 30 per cent wanted to limit their
families to two children, a mere 5 per cent favoring one or none.
The rest preferred at least three offspring.[4]

   The lack of support for voluntary sterilization has been
equally pronounced at all levels of government. Except for
Medicaid and recent OEO funds, Washington's family planning
programs never mention it. Only a handful of states like Colorado and Tennessee include sterilization in their funds for birth
control. "Planning for a Family," the recent lavish brochure of
New York City's Human Resources Administration, never refers to sterilization in 24 pages!

   Whether for the benefit of an individual who has decided
to have no more children, or for the nation as a whole whose survival demands rigorous population control, it seems obvious
that voluntary sterilization must become an integral part of public health policy. The intensifying public demand for both sterilization and legalized abortion has now brought us to the point
where zero population growth — each individual replacing himself with only one birth — may be an immediate possibility. The
number of unwanted births each year, estimated at 750,000-800,000

by Princeton University's Office of Population Research, may soon be diminished, or even checked, by the advances of legalized abortion.[5] Compared with a mere 14,000 or so in 1966, legal abortions in 1971 may reach 400,000 (with a considerable number of others still being done secretly).

While abortion eliminates the desperate possibility of a specific unwanted birth, and contraception provides only daily protection with all the risks of nonuse and failure, sterilization has a unique and more potent role. Its overwhelming advantage is permanence and dependability. It prevents all births during the remainder of an individual's fertile life. Therefore, it becomes an especially superior technique for stabilizing population — a technique that must be promoted by medical and governmental policy if we are to come to grips immediately with our last real chance to achieve zero population growth.

The combined impact of our soaring rates of sterilization and legalized abortion (which together may prevent 2 million potential births annually if we include secret abortions) gives us the chance to duplicate the remarkable demographic achievement of Japan. (With about one million abortions annually since 1958, Japan slashed its birth rate in half, and has kept it there for the last decade.) Since each sterilization, particularly among young couples, contributes far more to population control than each abortion, our paramount objective today must be a massive sterilization campaign, focused on couples under age 30, so that the chance of an unwanted pregnancy in the remaining 15 or 20 years of a woman's fertility can be eliminated.

This is the critical group today — young women and their husbands in their twenties, born during the "baby boom" after World War II. If this dangerously large group of potential parents decides to have more than two children per couple, they could send the U. S. birth rate into another spiraling cycle. But if they limit their offspring to two or less, and maintain this limit through sterilization, we may reach the turning point in population control.

A truly effective sterilization campaign would demand exhaustive financing and coordination on all federal and state levels. As John D. Rockefeller III, chairman of the Population

Council, has pointed out, "The problems of population are so great, so important, so ramified, and often so immediate that only government, supported and inspired by private initiative, can attack them on the scale required. . . ." Impressive as the expansion in vasectomy clinics had been in the last two years, a total attack requires that male and female sterilization clinics be available in every neighborhood so that no one would have to search or undergo inconvenient and expensive travel to find a facility. Sterilization as well as abortion would be offered free as a public health measure.

The achievement of zero population in the next decade would also necessitate a revolutionary restructuring of social thinking. The orientation of young couples towards sterilization would have to begin in high school and college as part of a coordinated program of sex education. Equally important is the promotion of a new feminist concept of the American family — a guarantee to women of equal opportunity in careers, education, and community service so that their happiness and fulfillment outside the home will persuade an increasing number to limit their offspring to one or two, and then embark at an early age on new interests beyond childbearing.

An essential step would be federal laws to give women equal job opportunity and pay, and enable them to compete with men as corporation executives as well as bookkeepers. A network of day care centers in every neighborhood would also have to be provided to allow mothers with young children to work or study outside the home. Discriminatory taxation must be revised so that rates no longer penalize single persons (who now pay more than married persons of equivalent income). If an overpopulated society benefits from a childless single man or woman, they should be rewarded rather than punished by the tax system.

The great challenge of our time is whether zero population growth can be achieved by such voluntary persuasion. And more important, whether it can be achieved fast enough. The frightening result of delay appears in statistical projections by Dr. Thomas Frejka of the Population Council. If it takes 50 years for all families to accept the two-child limit, our population in the meantime would probably double to about 400 millions! Can we delay that long with voluntary half-measures "while the human race proceeds apace towards breeding and starving itself into oblivion," as Associate Editor Tom Wicker of *The New York Times* describes the alternative.

Or have we the courage to grapple with the crisis now and accept the dictum that "having a child is no longer a matter of private will, but of public welfare," as Dr. Ashley Montagu, the noted anthropologist, has put it. "Whatever endangers the public welfare should, therefore, be carefully regulated."

No one welcomes the imposition of compulsory controls. Yet, why is it so hard to accept controls over birth when we have always accepted death control? In fact, life extension through public health programs (cutting the number of deaths to one for about every two births in the world) and the prolongation of terminal illness for months and years, often against the patient's will, are partly responsible for our exploding population.

One form of moderate control would be to raise the minimum age of marriage by law to 22 or 23. By diminishing hasty marriages at an early age, couples would tend to plan their children more carefully. While premarital pregnancies might increase, legalized abortion would probably allow most of these pregnancies to be terminated.

An even more effective second step in controls would be economic penalties against couples who bear three or more children — a sharp tax on the third, even heavier taxes on the fourth or succeeding births. Since penalties must not discriminate against any economic, social, or racial group, particularly the poor, they would have to be based on graduated income. A family with a $6,000 income, for example, might be taxed $600 for a third child while a family with $50,000 would pay $15,000.

The great advantage of such economic penalties is that they would stimulate the trend towards voluntary sterilization. A couple which now favors a two-child limit, but decides to adjust to a third pregnancy, often accidental and unwanted, would be sharply motivated by this heavy tax to make an immediate choice of abortion, and then eliminate any future pregnancy through sterilization. Most couples today are impelled towards sterilization by the threat of years of inconvenient and unpalatable contraception. If this threat is intensified by economic penalty, they would undoubtedly make their decision for sterilization at an earlier age.

Once most Americans have gotten over their psychological hangups over sterilization (their fears of impotence and other sexual damage long proved baseless by medical studies), the real block is to face the renunciation of fertility. The possible death of a living child, or a spouse's death and the survivor's remarriage, makes us cling to fertility as if it encompassed our own immortality. The development of sperm banks, and the rapid strides towards reversible sterilization should soon alleviate this primordial trauma. We are also learning that biological reproduction is not the only form of immortality or family life. An increasing number of couples are adopting children after one or two biological children, and finding they can fulfill their parental instincts with foster care, part-time summer adoptions, and volunteer service at day care and education centers.

The terrifying threat of population havoc presents an irrefutable incentive towards sterilization. If we have to give up the right to bear a third or fourth child, we are preserving the greater freedom of sanity and survival. Without a two-child limit, the present chaos of over-crowded schools and highways, the pollution of our air and environment will soon accelerate to a nightmare existence in 100-story apartment and business complexes where we would travel through air-conditioned, underground tunnels, and only venture on the streets with breathing masks. Normal luxuries like beef would be rationed once a month, parks and play space would be gobbled up for new construction, and transportation so controlled we would have to get a permit months ahead to visit another city. "If the world population continues to increase at the same rate, we will destroy the species," Dr. Norman E. Borlaug, winner of the 1970 Nobel Peace Prize and "Green Revolution" agronomist, reminds us.

1. *Chicago Tribune,* February 20, 1971.
2. Susan C. Scrimshaw and Bernard Pasquariella, "Variables Associated with the Acceptance of Surgical Sterilization Among Women in Spanish Harlem," International Institute for the Study of Reproduction, Columbia University, January 1970.
3. "Role of Female Sterilization in Population Control," *American Journal of Obstetrics & Gynecology,* Vol. 101, No. 3, June 1, 1968, p. 351.
4. Thomas Eisner, Ari Van Tienhoven, Frank Rosenblatt, *Science,* January 23, 1970.
5. Leslie Aldridge Westoff and Charles F. Westoff, *From Now to Zero,* Boston: Little, Brown, 1971.

Notes on Contributors

Dugald Baird, M.D., is a member of the Medical Research Council and practices in the Sociology Research Unit of the University of Aberdeen, Scotland. He is the author of *Combined Textbooks of Obstetrics and Gynecology.*

Robert B. Benjamin, M.D., is a surgeon at the St. Louis Park Medical Center, Minneapolis, Minnesota.

W. P. Black, M.D., is a consultant obstetrician and gynecologist to the Glasgow Royal Infirmary, Scotland.

Joseph E. Davis, M.D., is a clinical assistant professor of urology, New York Medical College, and the president of the Association for Voluntary Sterilization, New York City.

Anselma Dell'Olio is a charter member of the National Organization for Women (NOW) and the founder and director of the New Feminist Theater.

Donald J. Dodds, M.D., is a former president of Planned Parenthood of Toronto.

Ernest Dunbar is a former senior editor of *Look Magazine.*

Helen Edey, M.D., is chairman of the Executive Committee of the Association for Voluntary Sterilization, New York City.

Carl B. Erling, M.D., is a general practitioner in St. Paul, Minnesota.

Andrew S. Ferber, M.D., practices medicine in the Family Studies section of the Bronx State Hospital, New York.

Matthew Freund, Ph.D., is professor of pharmacology and an associate professor of obstetrics and gynecology at New York Medical College.

Jeremiah S. Gutman is an attorney with the Civil Liberties Union.

Jaroslav F. Hulka, M.D., is an associate professor of obstetrics and gynecology at the University of North Carolina School of Medicine, Chapel Hill.

José L. Janer, M.Sc., has worked for Planned Parenthood in Puerto Rico.

Judson T. Landis is professor of family sociology at the University of California, Berkeley, and a co-author of *Building a Successful Marriage* and *Building Your Life.*

Abel J. Leader, M.D., is medical director of Planned Parenthood of Houston and a clinical professor of urology at Baylor College of Medicine.

Sarah Lewit is a research associate at the Bio-Medical Division of the Population Council and co-editor of *Advances in Planned Parenthood, 1965.*

Fredelle Maynard is a free-lance writer.

Lonny Myers, M.D., is former vice-president of the National Association for Repeal of Abortion Laws and directs a vasectomy clinic at Chicago's Midwest Population Center.

Robert S. Neuwirth, M.D., is director of the department of obstetrics and gynecology at the Bronx-Lebanon Hospital Center, New York, and an associate professor of obstetrics and gynecology at Columbia University College of Physicians and Surgeons.

Manuel E. Paniagua, M.D., has long been active in Planned Parenthood in Puerto Rico.

Kenneth H. Phillips is an educational planning and fund-raising specialist at the Institute of International Education in New York City.

Harriet F. Pilpel is legal counsel for the Association for Voluntary Sterilization, New York, and has represented the birth control movement for many years in its most significant cases. She is a co-author of *Your Marriage and the Law.*

Shirley B. Poffenberger is a free-lance writer and research assistant.

Thomas Poffenberger is an associate professor of education and population planning at the University of Michigan School of Public Health.

Harriet B. Presser is a demographer at the International Institute for the Study of Human Reproduction, Columbia University, and an associate professor of sociology at Livingston College, Rutgers University, New Jersey.

John R. Rague is Executive Director of the Association for Voluntary Sterilization, New York City.

A. B. Sclare is a consultant psychiatrist at the Eastern District Hospital, Glasgow, Scotland.

Matthew Tayback, Sc.D., is Assistant Secretary of Health, Baltimore, Maryland.

Barbara Thompson is associated with the University of Aberdeen, Scotland.

Christopher Tietze, M.D., is associate director at the Bio-Medical Division of the Population Council, New York City.

José L. Vázquez, M.A., has worked for Planned Parenthood in Puerto Rico.

Curtis Wood, Jr., M.D., has retired from his practice in obstetrics and gynecology in Ft. Washington, Pa. to become a full-time medical consultant to the Association for Voluntary Sterilization, New York City.

Evan McLeod Wylie is a free-lance writer.

Appendix I

Vasectomy Clinics Currently Operating
in the United States as of November 1, 1971

Prepared by

ASSOCIATION FOR VOLUNTARY STERILIZATION, INC.

14 West 40th Street, New York, New York   10018

(Note: The names of the following facilities were obtained from diverse sources. Sometimes there is conflicting information about the program of a particular facility. Cross-checks with reliable local informants are recommended to be sure what services are currently provided.)

ALASKA
Anchorage Community Hospital*
825 L Street
Anchorage, Alaska   99501

ARIZONA
Planned Parenthood Assoc. of Phoenix
1200 South Fifth Avenue
Phoenix, Arizona   85003

Pima County Health Department
Pima County General Hospital
2900 South Sixth Avenue
Tucson, Arizona   85713

Planned Parenthood of Tucson
127 South Fifth Avenue
Tucson, Arizona   85701

Tucson Medical Center*
Grant Road at Beverly
Tucson, Arizona   85712

CALIFORNIA
Delta Memorial Hospital*
3901 Lone Tree Way, Box 236
Antioch, California   94509

Alta Bates Community Hospital*
Webster at Regent
Berkeley, California   94705

Herrick Hospital*
2001 Dwight Way
Berkeley, California   94704

American River Health Care Center*
4747 Engle Road
Carmichael, California   95608

Eden Hospital*
20103 Lake Chabot Road
Castro Valley, California   94546

Laurel Grove Hospital*
19933 Lake Chabot Road
Castro Valley, California   94546

*Vasectomy being performed in Out-Patient Department.

Concord Community Hospital*
2540 East Street
Concord, California   94520

Fresno Community Hospital*
Fresno and R Streets
Fresno, California   93720

Glendale Adventist Hospital*
1509 East Wilson Street
Glendale, California   91206

Planned Parenthood-World Population
  Alameda-San Francisco
Hayward Branch Vas Clinic
Hayward, California

Lakeside Community Hospital*
Lakeshore Drive
Lakeport, California   95453

Scripps Memorial Hospital*
9888 Genessee Avenue, Box 28
La Jolla, California   92037

Planned Parenthood-World Population
3100 West 8th Street
Los Angeles, California   90005

UCLA Medical Center
10833 Le Conte Avenue
Los Angeles, California   90024

White Memorial Medical Center*
1700 Brooklyn Avenue
Los Angeles, California   90033

Women's Hospital*
USC Medical Center
1240 North Mission Road
Los Angeles, California   90033

Contra Costa County Medical Services
(Out-patient clinics in
  Richmond & Pittsburgh)
2500 Alhambra Avenue
Martinez, California   94553

Martinez Community Hospital*
20 Allen Street, Box 991
Martinez, California   94553

El Camino Hospital*
2500 Grant Road
Mountain View, California   94040

Highland General Hospital*
1411 E. 31st Street
Oakland, California   94602

Stanford University Hospital*
300 Pasteur Drive
Palo Alto, California   94304

Kaiser Foundation Hospital*
13652 Cantara Street
Panorama City, California   91402

Pittsburg Community Hospital
550 School Street
Pittsburg, California   94565

Kaiser Foundation Hospital*
So. 14th Street & Cutting Blvd.
Richmond, California   94804

Richmond Hospital*
23rd Street & Gaynor Avenue
Richmond, California   94804

Parkview Community Hospital*
3865 Jackson Avenue
Riverside, California   92503

Sacramento Medical Center*
2315 Stockton Blvd.
Sacramento, California   95817

Sutter Memorial Hospital*
52nd and F Streets
Sacramento, California   95819

Kaiser Foundation Hospital*
2425 Geary Boulevard
San Francisco, California   94115

San Francisco General*
1001 Potrero Avenue
San Francisco, California   94110

Harold D. Chope Community Hospital
222 West 39th Avenue
San Mateo, California   94403

San Mateo Planned Parenthood Vas Clinic
45 No. "B" Street
San Mateo, California   94401

Brookside Hospital*
Vale Road
San Pablo, California   94806

Marin General Hospital*
250 Bon Air Road
Box 2129
San Rafael, California   94901

Los Angeles County
Harbor General Hospital*
1000 West Carson Street
Torrance, California   90502

John Muir Hospital*
Ygnacio Valley Road
Walnut Creek, California   94598

Kaiser Foundation Hospital*
1425 So. Main Street
Walnut Creek, California   94596

COLORADO

Memorial Hospital*
1400 E. Boulder Street
Colorado Springs, Colorado   80909

Denver General Hospital Vas Clinic
West Sixth Avenue & Cherokee Street
Denver, Colorado   '80204

General Rose Memorial Hospital*
1050 Clermont Street
Denver, Colorado   80220

CONNECTICUT

Planned Parenthood League
of Connecticut
406 Orange Street
New Haven, Connecticut 06511

DISTRICT OF COLUMBIA

Freedman's Hospital*
6th & Bryant Street, N.W.
Washington, D. C.   20001

FLORIDA

Broward General Medical Center*
1600 South Andrews Avenue
Fort Lauderdale, Florida   33316

Memorial Hospital*
3501 Johnson Street
Hollywood, Florida   33021

Duval County Family Planning Project
(Planned Parenthood of N.E. Florida refers)
2255 Phyllis Street — Suite 101
Jacksonville, Florida   32204

Lee Davis Health Center
Hillsborough County Health Dept.
2313 E. 28th Avenue
Tampa, Florida

Palm Beach Family Life Services, Inc.
Medical Arts Building
1717 North Flagler Drive
West Palm Beach, Florida

GEORGIA

Kennestone Hospital*
Church Street
Marietta, Georgia   30060

ILLINOIS

Northwest Suburban Vasectomy Clinic
1430 North Arlington Heights Road
Arlington Heights, Illinois   60004

Cook County Hospital
Fantus Out-Patient Vasectomy Clinic
1825 West Harrison Street
Chicago, Illinois   60612

Midwest Population Center
100 East Ohio Street
Chicago, Illinois   60611

Planned Parenthood of Chicago
185 North Wabash Avenue
Chicago, Illinois   60601

Decatur Memorial Hospital*
2300 N. Edward Street, Box 2207
Decatur, Illinois   62526

Sherman Hospital*
Center Street
Elgin, Illinois   60120

INDIANA

Planned Parenthood of North
Central Indiana
Memorial Hospital Vas Clinic
615 N. Michigan Street
South Bend, Indiana   46601

Planned Parenthood of Vigo County
1024 South 6th Street
Terre Haute, Indiana   47807

IOWA

Sartori Memorial Hospital*
6th and College
Cedar Falls, Iowa   50613

University of Iowa Hospitals
  and Clinics*
Newton Road
Iowa City, Iowa   52240

Allen Memorial Hospital*
1825 Logan Avenue
Waterloo, Iowa   50703

Schoitz Memorial Hospital*
Ridgeway and Kimball Avenues
Waterloo, Iowa   50702

KENTUCKY

Northern Kentucky Family
  Planning Project
Division of Maternal and Child Health
315 East 15th Street
Covington, Kentucky   41011

Ephraim McDowell Hospital*
217 South Third Street
Danville, Kentucky   40422

Harlan Appalachian Regional Hospital*
Martins Fork Road
Box 960
Harlan, Kentucky   40831

University of Kentucky Medical Center
800 Rose Street
Lexington, Kentucky   40506
(Contact: Planned Parenthood
  of Lexington
331 W. Second Street
Lexington, Kentucky   40507)

Jewish Hospital*
217 East Chestnut Street
Louisville, Kentucky   40202

Methodist Hospital*
315 East Broadway
Louisville, Kentucky   40202

MARYLAND

Peoples Free Medical Clinic
3028 Greenmount Avenue
Baltimore, Maryland   21218

Planned Parenthood Assoc. of Maryland
517 North Charles Street
Baltimore, Maryland

Johns Hopkins Hospital*
601 North Broadway
Baltimore, Maryland   21205

Sinai Hospital, Inc.*
Belvedere Avenue at Green Spring
Baltimore, Maryland   21215

MASSACHUSETTS

Boston Family Planning Project
  Vasectomy Clinic
14 Porter Street
East Boston, Massachusetts

Health, Inc.
332 Longwood Avenue
Boston, Massachusetts

Marlboro Hospital*
57 Union Street
Marlboro, Massachusetts   01752

Waltham Hospital*
Hope Avenue
Waltham, Massachusetts   02154

Memorial Hospital*
119 Belmont Street
Worcester, Massachusetts   01605

MICHIGAN

The Washtenaw County League for
  Planned Parenthood
313 North First Street
Ann Arbor, Michigan   48103

Oakwood Hospital*
18101 Oakwood Boulevard
Dearborn, Michigan   48124

Planned Parenthood League, Inc.
Professional Plaza Concourse Bldg.
3750 Woodward Avenue
Detroit, Michigan   48201

Planned Parenthood Assoc.
  of Kent County
425 Cherry S.E.
Grand Rapids, Michigan   49502

Foote Memorial Hospital*
East Street
Jackson, Michigan

Tri-County Family Planning Clinic
Suite 405
701 North Logan Street
Lansing, Michigan   48915

Oakland Center Hospital*
P. O. Box 309
120 W. Eleven Mile Road
Royal Oak, Michigan   48068

South Haven Community Hospital*
South Bailey Avenue
South Haven, Michigan   49090

MINNESOTA
Glenwood Hills Hospital*
3901 Golden Valley Road
Golden Valley, Minnesota   55422

Hennepin County General Hospital*
Fifth and Portland
Minneapolis, Minnesota   55415

St. Paul-Ramsey Hospital and
  Medical Center
University at Jackson Street
St. Paul, Minnesota   55101

MISSISSIPPI
University of Mississippi Medical
  Center*
2500 North State Street
Jackson, Mississippi   39216

MISSOURI
Washington University School of
  Medicine
Wohl Hospital Building, Barnes
  Hospital Complex
4960 Audubon Avenue
St. Louis, Missouri   63110

MONTANA
Planned Parenthood of Missoula County
Room 213, Health Dept. Courthouse
  Annex
Missoula, Montana   59801

NEBRASKA
Family Planning Center
3830 Adams
Lincoln, Nebraska   68504

NEVADA
Sunrise Hospital*
3186 Maryland Parkway
Las Vegas, Nevada   89109

NEW HAMPSHIRE
Mary Hitchcock Memorial Hospital*
2 Maynard Street
Hanover, New Hampshire   03755

NEW JERSEY
Atlantic City Hospital*
1925 Pacific Avenue
Atlantic City, New Jersey   08401

Valley Hospital*
Linwood and North Van Dien Avenues
Ridgewood, New Jersey   07451

Shore Memorial Hospital*
New York and Sunny Avenues
Somers Point, New Jersey   08244

Cooper Hospital*
6th and Stevens Streets
Camden, New Jersey   08103

Cherry Hill Medical Center*
Chapel Avenue & Coopers Landing Road
Cherry Hill, New Jersey   08034

John F. Kennedy Community Hospital*
James Street
Edison, New Jersey   08817

Elizabeth General Hospital & Dispensary*
925 East Jersey Street
Elizabeth, New Jersey   07201

New Jersey Center for Infertility
485 Route 9W
Englewood Cliffs, New Jersey   07632

Paul Kimball Hospital*
600 River Avenue
Lakewood, New Jersey   08701

Monmouth Medical Center*
300 Second Avenue
Long Branch, New Jersey   07740

Morris Area Planned Parenthood
(Vas Clinic located in Dover,
  New Jersey)
197 Speedwell
Morristown, New Jersey   07960

Burlington County Memorial Hospital*
175 Madison Avenue
Mount Holly, New Jersey   08060

Jersey Shore Medical Center (Fitkin)*
1945 Corlies Avenue
Neptune, New Jersey   07753

Montclair Community Hospital*
120 Harrison Avenue
Montclair, New Jersey   07042

New Jersey College of Medicine &
  Dentistry*
Martland Hospital Unit
65 Bergen Street
Newark, New Jersey   07107

United Hospitals Medical Center*
15 South 9th Street
Newark, New Jersey   07107

Barnert Memorial Hospital Center*
680 Broadway
Paterson, New Jersey   07514

Princeton Hospital*
253 Witherspoon Street
Princeton, New Jersey   08540

Salem County Memorial Hospital*
Woodstown Road
Salem, New Jersey   08079

Medical Center of Vineland*
2815 E. Chestnut Avenue
Vineland, New Jersey   08360

NEW MEXICO

Bernalillo County Planned Parenthood
  Assoc., Inc.
113 Montclaire, S.E.
Albuquerque, New Mexico

Bernalillo County Medical Center*
University of New Mexico School
  of Medicine
2211 Lomas Boulevard, N.E.
Albuquerque, New Mexico   87106

NEW YORK CITY

Abraham Jacobi Hospital*
G.U. Clinic
Pelham Parkway and Eastchester Road
Bronx, New York   10461

Downstate Medical Center
450 Clarkson Avenue
Brooklyn, New York   11203
  Attn: Dr. Robert E. Hackett

Williamsburg General Hospital*
757 Bushwick Avenue
Brooklyn, New York   11211

Bellevue Hospital Vasectomy Service
First Avenue and East 27th Street
New York, New York   10016

French Polyclinic Medical Center*
330 West 30th Street
New York, New York   10001

Margaret Sanger Research Bureau
  Vasectomy Service
17 West 6th Street
New York, New York   10011

Flower-Fifth Avenue Hospital*
106th Street and Fifth Avenue
New York, New York   10029

NEW YORK STATE

Albany Medical Center Hospital*
New Scotland Avenue
Albany, New York   12208

Nassau County Medical Center*
2201 Hempstead Turnpike
East Meadow, New York   11554

Charles E. Wilson Memorial Hospital*
33-57 Harrison Street
Johnson City, New York   13790

Nassau Hospital*
Second Street
Mineola, New York   11501

Northern Westchester Hospital*
E. Main Street
Mount Kisco, New York   10549

DeGraff Hospital*
445 Tremont Street
North Tonawanda, New York   14120

Genesee Hospital*
224 Alexander Street
Rochester, New York   14607

Highland Hospial of Rochester*
South Avenue and Bellevue Drive
Rochester, New York   14620

Rochester General Hospital*
1425 Portland Avenue
Rochester, New York   14621

Metropolitan Medical Associates
   Vasectomy Clinic
521 Main Street
Sparkill, New York   10976

Syosset Hospital*
225 Jericho Turnpike
Syosset, New York   11791

Strong Memorial Hospital of the
   University of Rochester*
260 Crittenden Boulevard
Rochester, New York   14620

Planned Parenthood of Syracuse
1120 East Genesee Street
Syracuse, New York

Upstate Medical Center*
750 East Adams Street
Syracuse, New York   13210

White Plains Hospital*
41 East Post Road
White Plains, New York   10601

NORTH CAROLINA
Stanly County Hospital*
North 4th Street
Albemarle, North Carolina   28001

Lenoir Memorial Hospital*
Rhodes Avenue and College Street
Kinston, North Carolina   28501

NORTH DAKOTA
Dakota Hospital*
South University Drive
Fargo, North Dakota   58102

Grand Forks Clinic*
Grand Forks, North Dakota   58201

Good Samaritan Hospital*
Williston, North Dakota   58801

OHIO
Vasectomy Services, Inc.
3333 Vine Street
Cincinnati, Ohio   45220

OKLAHOMA
Planned Parenthood
Family Planning
Cameron College
P. O. Box 6368
Lawton, Oklahoma

Norman Municipal Hospital*
901 North Porter Street, Box 1308
Norman, Oklahoma   73069

Hillcrest Medical Center*
11th at Utica
Tulsa, Oklahoma   74104

OREGON
Josephine General Hospital*
Grants Pass, Oregon   97526

Bess Kaiser Hospital*
5055 N. Greely Avenue
Portland, Oregon   97217

McKenzie-Willamette Hospital*
1460 G Street
Springfield, Oregon   97477

PENNSYLVANIA
Easton Hospital*
21st and Lehigh Streets
Easton, Pennsylvania   18042

Monroe County Planned Parenthood
   Association
P. O. Box 76
East Stroudsburg, Pennsylvania   18301

General Hospital of Monroe County*
East Brown Street
East Stroudsburg, Pennsylvania   18301

Lancaster General Hospital*
555 North Duke Street
Lancaster, Pennsylvania   17604

Hospital of the University of
  Pennsylvania*
106 Dulles Bldg.
3400 Spruce Street
Philadelphia, Pennsylvania   19104

Planned Parenthood Assoc. of
  S.E. Pennsylvania
1402 Spruce Street
Philadelphia, Pennsylvania   19102

Temple University Medical Center
3401 North Broad Street
Philadelphia, Pennsylvania   19140

Planned Parenthood of Pittsburgh
526 Penn Avenue
Pittsburgh, Pennsylvania   15222

Guthrie Clinic Ltd.*
Sayre, Pennsylvania   18840

RHODE ISLAND
Lying-In Hospital
50 Maude Street
Providence, Rhode Island   02908

Planned Parenthood of Rhode Island
47 Aborn Street
Providence, Rhode Island   02903

SOUTH CAROLINA
Charleston County Health Department
334 Calhoun Street
Charleston, South Carolina   29401

TENNESSEE
Erlanger Hospital*
Wiehl Street
Chattanooga, Tennessee   37403

Morristown Hamblen Hospital*
North High Street
Morristown, Tennessee   37814

TEXAS
Planned Parenthood of Dallas
3620 Maple Avenue
Dallas, Texas   75219

Providence Memorial Hospital*
1901 North Oregon
El Paso, Texas

South El Paso Hospital*
702 E. Paisano
El Paso, Texas

John Peter Smith Hospital Vas Clinic
Tarrant County Hospital District
1500 S. Main Street
Fort Worth, Texas   76104

Planned Parenthood of Houston
3512 Travis Street
Houston, Texas   77002

Ben Taub General Hospital
Harris County Hospital District
1502 Taub Loop
Houston, Texas   77025

VERMONT
Planned Parenthood of Vermont
19 Church Street, Room 8
Burlington, Vermont   05401

VIRGINIA
Fairfax Hospital*
3300 Gallows Road
Fairfax, Virginia   22046

WASHINGTON
Kadlec Methodist Hospital*
1005 Goethals Street
Richland, Washington   99352

Northwest Hospital*
1551 North 120th Street
Seattle, Washington   98133

Population Dynamics Vasectomy Service
3829 Aurora Avenue North
Seattle, Washington   98103

WEST VIRGINIA
Memorial Hospital
3200 Noyes Avenue, S.E.
Charleston, West Virginia   25304
  Attn: Dorothea Fee, R.N.

West Virginia University Hospital*
Morgantown, West Virginia   26506

WISCONSIN

Beaumont Clinic Ltd.*
1821 S. Webster Avenue
Green Bay, Wisconsin   54301

Planned Parenthood Assoc.
 of Milwaukee
536 West Wisconsin Avenue
Milwaukee, Wisconsin   53203

Plymouth Clinic*
1000 Eastern Avenue
Plymouth, Wisconsin   53073

ADDITIONALLY, THE FOLLOWING OUT-PATIENT SERVICES ARE OFFERED FOR FEMALE STERILIZATION

Memorial Hospital   L
1200 South Fifth Avenue
Phoenix, Arizona   85003

Surgicenter   L
(Drs. Loeffer and Pent)
1040 East McDowell Road)
Phoenix, Arizona

Marin General Hospital   (vaginal TL)
250 Bon Air Road
Box 2129
San Rafael, California   94902

Denver General Hospital   L
Family Planning Clinic
(Tibor Engel, M.D., Director)
West Sixth Avenue and Cherokee St.
Denver, Colorado   80204

Wilmington Medical Center   L
501 West 14th Street, Box 1668
Wilmington, Delaware   19899

Jackson Memorial Hospital (culdoscopy)
1700 N.W. 10th Avenue
Miami, Florida   33136

Bayfront Medical Center   L
701 Sixth Street South
St. Petersburg, Florida   33701

Michael Reese Hospital   L
2929 South Ellis Avenue
Chicago, Illinois   60616

Johns Hopkins Hospital   L
601 North Broadway
Baltimore, Maryland   21205

St. Luke's Hospital of
 Kansas City   L
Wornall Road at 44th Street
Kansas City, Missouri   64111

Miami Valley Hospital   L
1 Wyoming Street
Dayton, Ohio   45409

HEW Family Planning Project of
 Northeastern Oklahoma   L
Tulsa, Oklahoma

CLINICS IN THE OFFING

Planned Parenthood of San Diego Cty.
1369 B Street
San Diego, California   92101

Planned Parenthood-World Population
 Alameda-San Francisco
476 W. MacArthur Blvd.
Oakland, California   94609
(Expecting to open Vas Clinics in both
Oakland and San Francisco)

Hawaii Planned Parenthood Center
 Vasectomy Clinic
200 North Vineyard Building
Honolulu, Hawaii   96817

Wyandotte City Dept. of Health
619 Ann Avenue
Kansas City, Kansas   66101

L denotes sterilization by laparoscopy.

Planned Parenthood Association of
  Washington, Warren & Saratoga
  Counties
11 Little Street
Glens Falls, New York   12801

Toledo Planned Parenthood
217 15th Street
Toledo, Ohio   43624

Mt. Sinai Hospital
11 E. 100th Street
New York, New York   10029

North Carolina Memorial Hospital   L
University of North Carolina
Chapel Hill, North Carolina   27514

Caldwell County Health Dept.
Lenoir, North Carolina

Planned Parenthood Association of
  Miami Valley
1713 E. 3rd Street
Dayton, Ohio   45403

ZPG-Rapid City, South Dakota

Mt. Sinai Medical Center   L
948 North 12th Street
Milwaukee, Wisconsin   53233

Appendix II

**Hospitals with Liberal Policies for Female
Sterilization — as of July 1, 1971**

Prepared by

ASSOCIATION FOR VOLUNTARY STERILIZATION, INC.

14 West 40th Street, New York, New York   10018

ARIZONA
Tucson Medical Center
Grant & Beverly Roads
Box 6067
Tucson, Arizona   85716

CALIFORNIA
Alta Bates Community Hospital
Webster & Regent Streets
Berkeley, California   94705

Herrick Memorial Hospital
2001 Dwight Way
Berkeley, California   94704

Peninsula Community Hospital
1783 El Camino Real
Burlingame, California   94010

Parkwood Community Hospital
7011 Shoup Avenue
Canoga Park, California   91304

Eden Hospital
20103 Lake Chabot Road
Castro Valley, California   94546

Laurel Grove Hospital
19933 Lake Chabot Road
Castro Valley, California   94546

Fresno Community Hospital
Fresno & R Streets
Fresno, California   93721

Grossmont District Hospital
5555 Grossmont Center Drive, Box 158
La Mesa, California   92041

Cedars Sinai Medical Center
8720 Beverly Boulevard
Los Angeles, California   90048
(Cedars of Lebanon, Mount Sinai)

Los Angeles County-University of
    Southern California Medical Center
Women's Hospital
1240 North Mission Road
Los Angeles, California   90033

Contra Costa County Hospital
2500 Alhambra Avenue
Martinez, California

Martinez Community Hospital
20 Allen
Martinez, California

El Camino Hospital
2500 Grant Road
Mountain View, California   94040

Civic Center Hospital
390 40th Street
Oakland, California   94609

Stanford University Hospital
300 Pasteur Drive
Palo Alto, California   94304

Kaiser Foundation Hospital
13652 Cantara Street
Panorama City, California   91402

Pittsburg Community Hospital
550 School Street
Pittsburg, California   94565

Shasta General Hospital
2630 Hospital Lane
Redding, California   96001

Richmond Hospital
23rd And Gaynor Avenue
Richmond, California

Parkview Community Hospital
3865 Jackson Avenue
Riverside, California   92503

San Bernardino County
  General Hospital
780 East Gilbert Street
San Bernardino, California   92404

Kaiser Foundation Hospital
2425 Geary Boulevard
San Francisco, California   94115

Memorial Hospital of San Leandro
2800 Benedict Drive
San Leandro, California   94577

Brookside Hospital
2000 Vale Road
San Pablo, California   94806

Dameron Hospital
525 West Acacia
Stockton, California   95203

Kaiser Foundation Hospital
1425 South Main Street
Walnut Creek, California

John Muir Hospital
1601 Ygnacio Valley Road
Walnut Creek, California

COLORADO
Denver General Hospital
W. Sixth Avenue & Cherokee Street
Denver, Colorado   80204

General Rose Memorial Hospital
1050 Clermont St.
Denver, Colorado   80220

DISTRICT OF COLUMBIA
Columbia Hospital for Women
24th and L Streets, N.W.
Washington, D.C.   20037

Freedman's Hospital
6th and Bryant Streets, N.W.
Washington, D.C.   20001

Sibley Memorial Hospital
5255 Loughboro Road N.W.
Washington, D.C.   20016

Washington Hospital Center
110 Irving Street N.W.
Washington, D.C.   20010

FLORIDA
Broward General Medical Center
1600 S. Andrews Avenue
Fort Lauderdale, Florida   33316

Mt. Sinai Hospital of Greater Miami
4300 Alton Road
Miami Beach, Florida   33140

Tampa General Hospital
Davis Islands
Tampa, Florida   33606

GEORGIA
Athens General Hospital
797 Cobb Street
Athens, Georgia   30601

Kennestone Hospital
737 Church Street
Marietta, Georgia   30060

ILLINOIS
Central Community Hospital
5701 South Wood Street
Chicago, Illinois   60636

Michael Reese Hospital and
  Medical Center
2929 South Ellis Avenue
Chicago, Illinois   60616

Sydney R. Forkosh Memorial Hospital
2544 West Montrose Avenue
Chicago, Illinois   60618

Lake View Memorial Hospital
812 North Logan
Danville, Illinois   61832

Sherman Hospital
934 Center Street
Elgin, Illinois   60120

Highland Park Hospital
718 Glenview Avenue
Highland Park, Illinois   60035

INDIANA

Lutheran Hospital of Fort Wayne
3024 Fairfield Avenue
Fort Wayne, Indiana   46807

Community Hospital of Indianapolis
1500 North Ritter Avenue
Indianapolis, Indiana   46219

Union Hospital
1606 North 7th Street
Terre Haute, Indiana   47804

IOWA

University of Iowa Hospitals and Clinics
Newton Road
Iowa City, Iowa   52240

Saint Luke's Medical Center
2720 Stone Park Boulevard, Box 2000
Sioux City, Iowa   51104

KANSAS

Wesley Medical Center
550 North Hillside Avenue
Wichita, Kansas   67214

KENTUCKY

Ephraim McDowell Hospital
217 S. Third Street
Danville, Kentucky   40422

Central Baptist Hospital
1740 South Limestone Street
Lexington, Kentucky   40503

Good Samaritan Hospital
310 South Limestone Street
Lexington, Kentucky   40508

LOUISIANA

Highland Hospital
1006 Highland Avenue
Shreveport, Louisiana   71107

MARYLAND

Johns Hopkins Hospital
601 North Broadway Street
Baltimore, Maryland   21205

Sinai Hospital of Baltimore
Belvedere Avenue at Greenspring
Baltimore, Maryland   21215

Memorial Hospital
Memorial Avenue
Cumberland, Maryland   21502

MASSACHUSETTS

The Nashoba Community Hospital
15 Winthrop Avenue
Ayer, Massachusetts   01432

University Hospital
750 Harrison Avenue
Boston, Massachusetts   02118

Wesson Memorial Hospital
140 High Street
Springfield, Massachusetts   01105

MICHIGAN

Emma L. Bixby Hospital
818 Riverside Avenue
Adrian, Michigan   49221

University Hospital
140 S.E. Ann Street
Ann Arbor, Michigan   48104

Community Hospital
200 Tompkins Street
Battle Creek, Michigan   49106

Oakwood Hospital
18101 Oakwood Boulevard
Dearborn, Michigan   48124

W. A. Foote Memorial Hospital
205 N. East Avenue
Jackson, Michigan   49201

Oakland Center Hospital
P. O. Box 309
120 West Eleven Mile Road
Royal Oak, Michigan 48067

MINNESOTA
Glenwood Hills Hospital
3901 Golden Valley Road
Minneapolis, Minnesota 55422

Hennepin County General Hospital
Fifth and Portland Streets
Minneapolis, Minnesota 55415

Methodist Hospital
6500 Excelsior Boulevard
Saint Louis Park, Minnesota 55426

Rice Memorial Hospital
402 West 3rd Street
Willmar, Minnesota 56201

MISSISSIPPI
University Hospital
2500 North State Street
Jackson, Mississippi 39216

MISSOURI
University of Missouri Medical Center
807 Stadium Road
Columbia, Missouri 65201

Saint Luke's Hospital
Wornall Road & 44th Street
Kansas City, Missouri 64111

NEBRASKA
Bryan Memorial Hospital
4848 Summer Street
Lincoln, Nebraska 68506

Dodge County Hospital
450 East 23rd Street
Tremont, Nebraska 68025

NEVADA
Sunrise Hospital
3186 Maryland Parkway
Las Vegas, Nevada 89114

NEW JERSEY
Atlantic City Hospital
1925 Pacific Avenue
Atlantic City, New Jersey 08401

Englewood Hospital
350 Engle Street
Englewood, New Jersey 07631

Beth Israel Hospital
70 Parker Avenue
Passaic, New Jersey 07055

Barnert Memorial Hospital Center
680 Broadway
Paterson, New Jersey 07514

Valley Hospital
Linwood & North Van Dien Avenue
Ridgewood, New Jersey 07451

Shore Memorial Hospital
New York & Sunny Avenues
Somers Point, New Jersey 08244

NEW MEXICO
Bernalillo County Medical Center
2211 Lomas Boulevard N.E.
Albuquerque, New Mexico 87106

Las Vegas Hospital
1235 Eighth Street, Box 238
Las Vegas, New Mexico 87701

NEW YORK
Bronx Municipal Hospital Center
Pelham Parkway and Eastchester Road
Bronx, New York

Montefiore Hospital and Medical Center
111 East 210th Street
Bronx, New York 10467

Morrisania City Hospital
168th and Gerard Avenue
Bronx, New York 10452

Coney Island Hospital
Ocean & Shore Parkways
Brooklyn, New York 11235

State University Hospital
Downstate Medical Center
450 Clarkson Avenue
Brooklyn, New York 11203

Williamsburgh General Hospital
757 Bushwick Avenue
Brooklyn, New York 11221

Buffalo General Hospital
100 High Street
Buffalo, New York   14203

Children's Hospital
219 Bryant Street
Buffalo, New York   14222

Millard Fillmore Hospital
3 Gates Circle
Buffalo, New York   14209

Ideal Hospital of Endicott
600 High Avenue
Endicott, New York   13760

Huntington Hospital
270 Park Avenue
Huntington, New York   11743

Charles S. Wilson Memorial Hospital
33-57 Harrison Street
Johnson City, New York   13790

North Shore Hospital
Valley Road
Manhasset, New York   11030

Northern Westchester Hospital
East Main Street
Mount Kisco, New York   10549

Beth Israel Medical Center
10 Nathan D. Pearlman Place
New York, New York   10003

French & Polyclinic Medical School
  & Health Center
French Hospital Division
330 West 30th Street
New York, New York   10001

New York Polyclinic Hospital Division
345 West 50th Street
New York, New York   10019

Harlem Hospital Center
506 Lenox Avenue
New York, New York   10037

New York Medical College-Flower &
  Fifth Avenue Hospital
1249 Fifth Avenue
New York, New York   10029

The Roosevelt Hospital
428 West 59th Street
New York, New York   10019

Woman's Hospital of Saint Luke's
  Hospital Center
Amsterdam & 114th Street
New York, New York   10025

De Graff Memorial Hospital
445 Tremont Street
North Tonawanda, New York   14120

City Hospital Center at Elmhurst
79-01 Broadway
Elmhurst Station, Flushing
Queens, New York   11373

Highland Hospital of Rochester
South Avenue & Bellevue Drive
Rochester, New York   14620

Rome Hospital & Murphy Memorial
  Hospital
1500 North James Street
Rome, New York   13440

Staten Island Hospital
101 Castleton Avenue
Staten Island, New York   10301

Crouse-Irving Memorial Hospital
736 Irving Avenue
Syracuse, New York   13210

NORTH CAROLINA

Stanly County Hospital
North Fourth Street
Albemarle, North Carolina   28001

North Carolina Memorial Hospital
University of North Carolina
Chapel Hill, North Carolina   27514

Watts Hospital
Broad Street at Club Boulevard
Durham, North Carolina   27705

Onslow Memorial Hospital
Corner College & Warlick Streets, Box129
Jacksonville, North Carolina   28540

Lenoir Memorial Hospital
Rhodes Avenue & College Street
Kinston, North Carolina   28501

NORTH DAKOTA

Dakota Hospital
1720 South University Drive
Fargo, North Dakota   58102

OHIO

Jane M. Case Hospital
561 West Central Avenue
Delaware, Ohio   43015

Hardin Memorial Hospital Company
921 East Franklin Street
Kenton, Ohio   43326

OKLAHOMA

Norman Municipal Hospital
901 North Porter Street, Box 1308
Norman, Oklahoma   73069

OREGON

Josephine General Hospital
715 N.W. Dimmick Street
Grants Pass, Oregon   97526

Bess Kaiser Hospital
5055 North Greely Avenue
Portland, Oregon   97217

Tillamook County General Hospital
1000 Third Street
Tillamook, Oregon   97141

PENNSYLVANIA

United Hospital
900 Third Avenue
Beaver Falls, Pennsylvania   15010

Easton Hospital
21st & Lehigh Streets
Easton, Pennsylvania   18042

General Hospital of Monroe County
206 East Brown Street
East Stroudsburg, Pennsylvania   18301

Lancaster General Hospital
555 North Duke Street
Lancaster, Pennsylvania   17604

Albert Einstein Medical Center
York & Tabor Roads
Philadelphia, Pennsylvania   19141

Frankford Hospital of the City of
    Philadelphia
Frankford Avenue & Wakeling Street
Philadelphia, Pennsylvania   19124

Hospital of the University of Pennsylvania
3400 Spruce Street
Philadelphia, Pennsylvania   19104

Jeanes Hospital
Hartel & Hasbrook Streets
Philadelphia, Pennsylvania   19111

Presbyterian-University of Pennsylvania
    Medical Center
51 North 39th Street
Philadelphia, Pennsylvania   19104

Temple University Hospital
3401 North Broad Street
Philadelphia, Pennsylvania   19140

Western Pennsylvania Hospital
4800 Friendship Avenue
Pittsburgh, Pennsylvania   15224

Magee Women's Hospital
Forbes Avenue & Halket Street
Pittsburgh, Pennsylvania   15213

RHODE ISLAND

Providence Lying-In Hospital
50 Maude Street
Providence, Rhode Island   02908

TENNESSEE

Morristown-Hamblen Hospital
727 West Fourth North Street
Morristown, Tennessee   37814

Lauderdale County Hospital
Tucker Avenue
Ripley, Tennessee   38063

TEXAS

South El Paso Hospital
702 East Paisano Drive
El Paso, Texas   79901

Valley Baptist Hospital
2101 South Commerce Street, Box 2588
Harlingen, Texas   78550

VERMONT

Medical Center Hospital of Vermont
Colchester Avenue
Burlington, Vermont   05401

WASHINGTON

Northwest Hospital
1551 North 120th Street
Seattle, Washington   98133

Swedish Hospital Medical Center
1212 Columbia Street
Seattle, Washington   98104

WEST VIRGINIA
West Virginia University Hospital
Morgantown, West Virginia   26500

WISCONSIN
Kenosha Memorial Hospital
6308 Eighth Avenue
Kenosha, Wisconsin   53140

Plymouth Hospital
210 Selma Street
Plymouth, Wisconsin   53073

Appendix III

**Hospitals Where Female Sterilization
Is Performed — as of July 1, 1971**

Prepared by

ASSOCIATION FOR VOLUNTARY STERILIZATION, INC.

14 West 40th Street, New York, New York   10018

Laparoscopy

ARIZONA
Memorial Hospital
1200 South Fifth Avenue
Phoenix, Arizona   85003

CALIFORNIA
Alta Bates Community Hospital
Webster & Regent Streets
Berkeley, California   94705

Cedars-Sinai Medical Center
Cedars of Lebanon Hospital Division
4833 Fountain Avenue
Los Angeles, California   90029

Mt. Sinai Hospital Division
8720 Beverly Boulevard
Los Angeles, California   90048

Brookside Hospital
2000 Vale Road
San Pablo, California   94806

Dameron Hospital
525 W. Acacia Street
Stockton, California   95203

San Antonio Community Hospital
999 San Bernardino Road
Upland, California   91786

COLORADO
Denver General Hospital
West 6th Avenue & Cherokee Street
Denver, Colorado   80204

CONNECTICUT
Hartford Hospital
80 Seymour Street
Hartford, Connecticut   06115

DELAWARE
Wilmington Medical Center
501 West 14th Street, Box 1668
Wilmington, Delaware   19899

DISTRICT OF COLUMBIA
Columbia Hospital for Women
2425 L Street, N.W.
Washington, D.C.   20037

George Washington University Hospital
901 23rd Street, N.W.
Washington, D.C. 20037

Washington Hospital Center
110 Irving Street, N.W.
Washington, D.C. 20010

FLORIDA

University of Florida Medical School
Gainesville, Florida 32601

Baptist Memorial Hospital
800 Miami Road
Jacksonville, Florida 32207

Methodist Hospital
1640 Jefferson Street
Jacksonville, Florida 32204

University Hospital
(formerly Duval Medical Center)
2000 Jefferson Street
Jacksonville, Florida 32206
(Box 2751, West Bay Annex 32203)

Lakeland General Hospital
Lakeland Hills Boulevard
Lakeland, Florida 33802

Palm Beach Gardens
Community Hospital
3360 Burns Road
Palm Beach, Florida 33480

Bayfront Medical Center
701 Sixth Street South
St. Petersburg, Florida 33701

St. Petersburg General Hospital
6500 38th Avenue North
St. Petersburg, Florida 33710

Tampa General Hospital
Davis Islands
Tampa, Florida 33606

GEORGIA

Memorial Medical Center
Waters Avenue at 63rd Street
Box 6688 Station C
Savannah, Georgia 31405

ILLINOIS

Michael Reese Hospital
2929 South Ellis Avenue
Chicago, Illinois 60616

University of Chicago Hospitals & Clinics
Chicago Lying-In Hospital
950 East 59th Street
Chicago, Illinois 60637

Hinsdale Sanitarium and Hospital
120 North Oak Street
Hinsdale, Illinois 60521

Community Memorial General Hospital
5101 Wilson Springs Road
La Grange, Illinois 60525

Proctor Community Hospital
5409 North Knoxville Avenue
Peoria, Illinois 61614

Memorial Hospital of Springfield
First and Miller Streets
Springfield, Illinois 62701

Carle Foundation Hospital
611 West Park Street
Urbana, Illinois 61801

Victory Memorial Hospital
1324 North Sheridan Road
Waukegan, Illinois 60085

INDIANA

Community Hospital
1500 North Ritter
Indianapolis, Indiana 46219

KANSAS

University of Kansas Medical Center
39th Street and Rainbow Boulevard
Kansas City, Kansas 66103

Wesley Medical Center
550 North Hillside Avenue
Wichita, Kansas 67214

KENTUCKY

Louisville General Hospital
323 E. Chestnut Street
Louisville, Kentucky 40202

MARYLAND
Greater Baltimore Medical Center
6701 North Charles Street
Baltimore, Maryland   21204

Johns Hopkins Hospital
601 N. Broadway Street
Baltimore, Maryland   21205

Sinai Hospital of Baltimore
Belvedere Avenue at Greenspring
Baltimore, Maryland   21215

Montgomery General Hospital
2801 Olney-Sandy Spring Road
Olney, Maryland   20832 (D.C. area)

MASSACHUSETTS
Beth Israel Hospital
330 Brookline Avenue
Boston, Massachusetts   02215

Peter Bent Brigham Hospital
721 Huntington Avenue
Boston, Massachusetts   02115

MICHIGAN
University Hospital
1405 East Ann Street
Ann Arbor, Michigan   48104

Beyer Memorial Hospital
135 South Prospect Street
Ypsilanti, Michigan   48147

MINNESOTA
University of Minnesota Hospitals
412 Union Street, S.E.
Minneapolis, Minnesota   55455

MISSISSIPPI
University Medical Center
2500 N. State Street
Jackson, Mississippi   39216

MISSOURI
Independence Sanitarium and Hospital
1509 West Truman Road
Independence, Missouri   64050

Baptist Memorial Hospital
6601 Rockhill Road
Kansas City, Missouri   64131

Kansas City General Hospital
and Medical Center
24th and Cherry Streets
Kansas City, Missouri   64108

Research Hospital and Medical Center
Meyer Boulevard and Prospect Avenue
Kansas City, Missouri   64132

St. Luke's Hospital of Kansas City
Wornall Road at 44th St.
Kansas City, Missouri   64111

Barnes Hospital
Barnes Hospital Plaza
St. Louis, Missouri   63110

NEBRASKA
University Hospital, University of
Nebraska
42nd Street and Dewey Avenue
Omaha, Nebraska   68105

NEW YORK
Albany Medical Center
New Scotland Avenue
Albany, New York   12208

Bronx-Lebanon Hospital Center
1276 Fulton Ave.
Bronx, New York   10450

Albert Einstein College of Medicine
Municipal Hospital Center
Pelham Parkway and Eastchester Road
Bronx, New York   10461

Downstate Medical Center
450 Clarkson Avenue
Brooklyn, New York   11203

Deaconess Hospital
1001 Humbaldt Parkway
Buffalo, New York   14208

North Shore Hospital
Valley Road
Manhasset, New York   11034

LeRoy Hospital
40 East 61st Street
New York, New York,

New York Hospital — Lying-In
525 East 68th Street
New York, New York   10021

The Roosevelt Hospital
428 West 59th Street
New York, New York 10019

St. Luke's Hospital Center —
   Women's Hospital
Amsterdam and 114th Street
New York, New York 10025

Vassar Brothers Hospital
Reade Place
Poughkeepsie, New York 12601

Ellis Hospital
1101 Nott Street
Schnectady, New York 12308

NORTH CAROLINA

North Carolina Memorial Hospital
University of North Carolina
Chapel Hill, North Carolina 27514

OHIO

Miami Valley Hospital
1 Wyoming Street
Dayton, Ohio 45409

Charles F. Kettering Memorial Hospital
3535 Southern Boulevard
Kettering, Ohio 45429

Mansfield General Hospital
335 Glessner Avenue
Mansfield, Ohio 44903

Northside Hospital
Gypsy Lane and Goleta Avenue
Youngstown, Ohio 44501

OREGON

Emanuel Hospital
2801 North Gantenbein Avenue
Portland, Oregon 97227

PENNSYLVANIA

Frankford Hospital of the City of
   Philadelphia
Frankford Avenue and Wakeling Street
Philadelphia, Pennsylvania 19124

Hospital of the University of
   Pennsylvania
3400 Spruce Street
Philadelphia, Pennsylvania 19104

Pennsylvania Hospital
Eighth and Spruce Streets
Philadelphia, Pennsylvania 19107

Magee-Women's Hospital
Forbes Avenue & Halket Street
Pittsburgh, Pennsylvania 15213

St. Joseph's Hospital
215 North 12th Street
Reading, Pennsylvania 19603

SOUTH DAKOTA

Bennett-Clarkson Memorial Hospital
915 Mountain View Road
Rapid City, South Dakota 57701

TEXAS

Baylor Medical School
1200 Moursund Avenue
Houston, Texas 77025

VIRGINIA

Fairfax Hospital
3300 Gallows Road
Falls Church, Virginia 22046

Dixie Hospital
3120 Victoria Boulevard
Hampton, Virginia 23361

Norfolk General Hospital
600 Gresham Drive
Norfolk, Virginia 23507

Portsmouth General Hospital
900 Leckie Street
Portsmouth, Virginia 23704

Medical College of Virginia Hospitals
Virginia Commonwealth University
1200 East Broad Street
Richmond, Virginia 23219

WASHINGTON

Harborview Medical Center
325 Ninth Avenue
Seattle, Washington 98104

Northwest Hospital
1551 North 120th Street
Seattle, Washington 98113

Virginia Mason Hospital
1111 Terry Avenue
Seattle, Washington 98101

WISCONSIN

Mount Sinai Medical Center
948 North 12th Street
Milwaukee, Wisconsin   53233

Culdoscopy

Jackson Memorial Hospital
1700 N.W. 10th Avenue
Miami, Florida   33136

Johns Hopkins Hospital
601 North Broadway Street
Baltimore, Maryland   21205

Nebraska Methodist Hospital
8303 Dodge Street
Omaha, Nebraska   68114

LeRoy Hospital
40 East 61st Street
New York, New York

Appendix IV

Blue Cross-Blue Shield and Medicaid Insurance for Voluntary Sterilization — as of December 8, 1970

Prepared by:

ASSOCIATION FOR VOLUNTARY STERILIZATION, INC.
14 West 40th Street, New York, New York 10018

	BLUE CROSS		BLUE SHIELD			MEDICAID	
	Medical Necessity	Socio-Economic	Medical Necessity	Socio-Economic	Office Vasectomy	Medical Necessity	Socio-Economic
ALABAMA	Yes	Yes	Yes	Yes	Yes	Yes	No
ALASKA	NR	NR	NP	NP	NP	NP	NP
ARIZONA	No	No	No	No	No	NP	NP
ARKANSAS	Yes	Yes	Yes	Yes	Yes	Yes	Yes
CALIFORNIA (Hosp. Ser. of Cal., Oakland) Yes Yes (B.C. of So. Cal., L.A.) Most Some			Yes	No	Yes	Yes	No
COLORADO	Yes	Yes	Yes	Yes	Yes	Yes	No
CONN.	Yes	Yes	Yes	No	Yes	Yes	No
DELAWARE	Yes	Yes	Yes	Yes	Yes	Yes	Yes
D. C.	Yes	Yes	Yes	Yes	Yes	Yes	No
FLORIDA	NR	NR	NR	NR	NR	Yes	Yes
GEORGIA	Yes	Yes	Yes	Yes	Yes	Yes	Yes
HAWAII	NP	NP	No	No	No	Yes	Yes

NR means no reply   NP means no plan   NC means needs clarification

	BLUE CROSS		BLUE SHIELD			MEDICAID	
	Medical Necessity	Socio-Economic	Medical Necessity	Socio-Economic	Office Vasectomy	Medical Necessity	Socio-Economic
IDAHO	Yes	Yes	Yes	Yes	Yes	Yes	Yes
ILLINOIS	Yes	Yes	Yes	Yes	Yes	Yes	Yes
INDIANA	Yes	Yes	Yes	Yes	Yes	Yes	Yes
IOWA	Des Moines Yes Yes / Sioux City Yes No		Yes	Yes	Yes	Yes	Yes
KANSAS	Yes	Yes	Yes	Yes	Yes	Yes	Yes
KENTUCKY	Yes	Yes	Yes	Yes	Yes	Yes	Yes
LOUISIANA	Yes	Yes	NP	NP	NP	No	No
MAINE	Yes	Yes	Yes	Yes	Yes	Yes	Yes
MARYLAND	Yes	Yes	Yes	Yes	Yes	Yes	Yes
MASS.	Yes	No	Yes	No	Yes	Yes	No
MICHIGAN	Yes	Yes	Yes	No	No	Yes	Yes
MINNESOTA	Yes	Yes	Yes	Yes	No	Yes	Yes
MISSISSIPPI	Yes	Yes	Yes	Yes	Yes	Yes	Yes
MISSOURI	Yes	No	Yes	No	Yes	Yes	No
MONTANA	No, in general, but pays some.		No	No	No	Yes	Yes
NEBRASKA	NR	NR	NR	NR	NR	Yes	Yes
NEVADA	NP	NP	NP	NP	NP	Yes	Yes
NEW HAMPS.	Yes	Yes	Yes	Yes	Yes	Yes	Yes
NEW JERSEY	Yes	Yes	Yes	Yes	Yes	Yes	Yes
NEW MEXICO	Yes	Yes	Yes	Yes	Yes	Yes	No
NEW YORK	Yes	Yes	Yes	Yes	Yes	Yes	No
NO. CAR.	Yes	Yes	Yes	Yes	Yes	Yes	No
NO. DAK.	Yes	Yes	Yes	Yes	Yes	Yes	Yes
OHIO	Yes	Yes	Yes	Yes	Yes	Yes	NC
OKLAHOMA	Yes	Yes	Yes	Yes	Yes	Yes	Yes
OREGON	Yes	Yes	No	No	No	Yes	Yes
PENNSYLVANIA	Yes	Yes	Yes	Yes	Yes	Yes	Yes

NR means no reply   NP means no plan   NC means needs clarification

	BLUE CROSS		BLUE SHIELD			MEDICAID	
	Medical Necessity	Socio-Economic	Medical Necessity	Socio-Economic	Office Vasectomy	Medical Necessity	Socio-Economic
RHODE ISLAND	Yes	Yes	Yes	Yes	Yes	Yes	Yes
SO. CAROLINA	Yes	Yes	Yes	Yes	Yes	Yes	No
SO. DAKOTA	Yes	No	Yes	No	Yes	Yes	Yes
TENN.	Yes	Yes	Yes	Yes	Yes	Yes	Yes
TEXAS	Yes	Yes	Yes	Yes	Yes	Yes	Yes
UTAH	Yes	No	Yes	No	Yes	Yes	No
VERMONT	Yes	Yes	Yes	Yes	Yes	Yes	Yes
VIRGINIA	Yes	Yes	Yes	Yes	Yes	Yes	Yes
WASHINGTON	NR (One) (Plan)	NR	Of the 20 B.S. County and Regional Plans, some pay, some do not pay.			Yes	Yes
WEST VA.	Yes	Yes	Yes	Yes	Yes	Yes	No
WISCONSIN	NR	NR	Yes	No	No	Yes	No
WYOMING	NR	NR	NR	NR	NR	Yes	Yes
TOTAL STATES THAT PAY — INCLUDING D.C.	41	37	40 plus some D.C. plans	32 plus some D.C. plans	37 plus some D.C. plans	48	33

NR means no reply   NP means no plan   NC means needs clarification

NOTE: Blue Cross and Blue Shield information was compiled from replies to the following:

1. Does your company pay for voluntary sterilization operations when physician has indicated: a) A medical necessity for the operation?; b) A socio-economic need for the operation, and performed the operation on that basis?
2. Does your company pay for the male operation done in a physician's office?

Payments vary according to contracts.

Medicaid information was compiled from replies to the following:

1. Does your plan pay for voluntary sterilization when the physician indicates a medical necessity for the operation?
2. Does your plan pay for voluntary sterilization when the physician indicates a socio-economic need for the operation?

Grateful acknowledgment is made to the following for use of their material
in this book:

Robert Benjamin, M.D., for "Vasectomy as an Office Procedure," reprinted
with permission from the *Bulletin* of St. Louis Park Medical Center, Vol.
XIV, No. 1 (Winter 1970), pp. 13-25; W. P. Black, M.D., and A.B. Sclare
for "Sterilization by Tubal Ligation — A Follow-Up Study," reprinted with
permission from *The Journal of Obstetrics and Gynaecology of the British
Commonwealth,* Vol. 75 (February 1968), pp. 219-224; Donald J. Dodds,
M.D., for material reprinted with permission from *Voluntary Male Sterilization,*
copyright © 1970 by D. J. Dodds, M.D., and published by The Damion
Press, Toronto; Ernest Dunbar for "Foolproof Birth Control," reprinted with
permission from *Look Magazine* (March 9, 1971), © 1970 *Look Magazine;*
Helen Edey, M.D., for "Sterilization," reprinted with permission from *New
York Medicine* (August 1970); Carl B. Erling, M.D., for "One GP's Per-
sonal and Professional Commitment," reprinted with permission from
Medical Opinion (March 1971), p. 58; Andrew S. Ferber, M.D., Christopher
Tietze, M.D., and Sarah Lewit for "Men with Vasectomies: A Study of
Medical, Sexual, and Psychological Changes," reprinted by permission of
Harper & Row, Publishers, Inc. from *Psychosomatic Medicine,* Vol. XXIX,
No. 4 (July-August 1967), pp. 354-366, copyright © 1967 by Harper & Row
Publishers, Inc.; *Journal of American Medical Association* for "Voluntary
Male Sterilization," reprinted with permission from *JAMA,* Vol. 204, No. 9
(May 27, 1968); Judson T. Landis, M.D., and Thomas Poffenberger for
"Hesitations and Worries of 330 Couples," reprinted by permission of E. C.
Brown Trust Foundation, Portland, Oregon, from *Family Life Coordinator,*
Vol. XV, No. 4 (October 1966), pp. 143-47; Judson T. Landis, M.D., and
Thomas Poffenberger for "Marital and Sexual Adjustment of 330 Couples
Who Chose Vasectomy as a Form of Birth Control," reprinted with permission
from the *Journal of Marriage and the Family,* Vol. 27, No. 1 (February 1965),
pp. 57-58; Abel J. Leader, M.D., for "The Structure of a Large-Scale
Vasectomy Clinic," originally presented at the meeting of the American Asso-
ciation of Planned Parenthood Physicians in Kansas City, Mo. (April 1971),
and reprinted by permission of the American Association of Planned Parenthood
Physicians from *Advances in Planned Parenthood,* Vol. VII; Fredelle Maynard
for "At 22, My Husband Chose Sterilization," as told to Fredelle Maynard,
reprinted by permission of Curtis Brown, Ltd., from *Good Housekeeping*
(January 1971), copyright © 1970 by the Hearst Corporation; Manuel E.
Paniagua, M.D., Matthew Tayback, José L. Janer, and José Vázquez for
"Medical and Psychological Sequelae of Surgical Sterilization of Women,"
reprinted with permission from the *American Journal of Obstetrics and
Gynecology,* Vol. 90, pp. 421-30 (October 15, 1964), copyright 1964 The C. V.
Mosby Co., St. Louis, Mo.; Harriet F. Pilpel for "Know Your Rights about
Voluntary Sterilization"; Thomas Poffenberger and S. B. Poffenberger for
"Vasectomy as a Preferred Method of Birth Control," reprinted with permission from the *Journal of Marriage and the Family,* Vol. 25, No. 3 (August
1963), pp. 326-330; Harriet B. Presser for material reprinted by permission
of The Population Council from "Voluntary Sterilization: A World View,"
from *Reports on Population/Family Planning,* No. 5 (July 1970); The
Simon Population Trust for "Vasectomy: Follow-Up of One Thousand Cases,"
reprinted with permission from *The Simon Population Trust* (December 1969),

pp. 10-19; Barbara Thompson and Dugald Baird, M.D., for "Follow-Up of 186 Sterilized Women," reprinted with permission from *The Lancet* (May 11, 1968), pp. 1023-27; H. Curtis Wood, Jr., M.D., for "How to Meet and Survive a Wave of Demand," reprinted with permission from *Medical Opinion* (March 1970), p. 56; Evan M. Wylie for "Birth Control for Men," reprinted by permission of the International Famous Agency from *Reader's Digest* (January 1971), copyright © 1971 by The Reader's Digest Association; and for "New Birth-Control Freedom for Women," reprinted by permission of the International Famous Agency from *Reader's Digest* (August 1971), copyright © 1971 by The Reader's Digest Association.

Index